ISGE Series

Series Editor

Andrea R. Genazzani, Endocrinology, International Society of Gynecological
Endocrinology, Pisa, Italy

The ISGE Book Series is the expression of the partnership between the International Society of Gynecological Endocrinology and Springer. The book series includes single monographs devoted to gynecological endocrinology relevant topics as well as the contents stemming from educational activities run by ISGRE, the educational branch of the society. This series is meant to be an important tool for physicians who want to advance their understanding of gynecological endocrinology and master this difficult clinical area. The International Society of Gynecological ad Reproductive Endocrinology (ISGRE) School fosters education and clinical application of modern gynecological endocrinology throughout the world by organizing high-level, highly focused residential courses twice a year, the Winter and the Summer Schools. World renowned experts are invited to provide their clinical experience and their scientific update to the scholars, creating a unique environment where science and clinical applications melt to provide the definitive update in this continuously evolving field. Key review papers are published in the Series, thus providing a broad overview over time on the major areas of gynecological endocrinology.

Indexed in Scopus

- **Series Editor: Prof. Andrea R. Genazzani argenazzani@gmail.com**

Andrea R. Genazzani • Steven R. Goldstein
Tommaso Simoncini

Editors

Menstrual Bleeding and Pain Disorders from Adolescence to Menopause

Volume 11: Frontiers in Gynecological Endocrinology

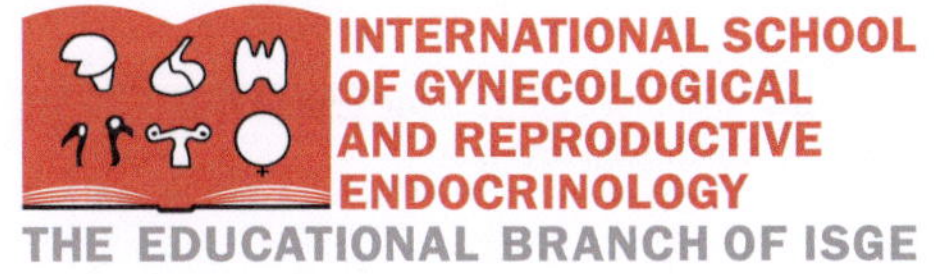

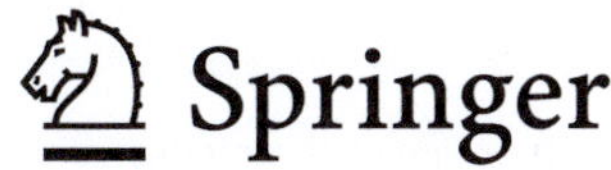

Editors
Andrea R. Genazzani
International Society of Gynecological
Endocrinology (ISGE)
Locarno, Switzerland

Steven R. Goldstein
Obstetrics and Gynecology
New York University Grossman
School of Medicine
New York, NY, USA

Tommaso Simoncini
Dept of Clinical & Experimental Medicine
University of Pisa
Pisa, Italy

ISSN 2197-8735   ISSN 2197-8743   (electronic)
ISGE Series
ISBN 978-3-031-55302-8   ISBN 978-3-031-55300-4   (eBook)
https://doi.org/10.1007/978-3-031-55300-4

This Springer imprint is published by the registered company Springer Nature Switzerland AG
The registered company address is: Gewerbestrasse 11, 6330 Cham, Switzerland

If disposing of this product, please recycle the paper.

Contents

About the Editors

Andrea R. Genazzani is Full Professor of Obstetrics and Gynecology and nominated Director of the Department of Obstetrics and Gynecology at the University of Cagliari. From 1° November 1982 he was nominated Director of the Department of Obstetrics and Gynecology at the University of Modena, and from 1994 to 2012 he served as the Director of the Department of Obstetrics and Gynecology at the University of Pisa. In 1994 he was awarded with the Honoris Causa Laurea by the University of Wroclaw (Poland), in 2005 by the University "Ovidius" of Costanta (Romania), in 2007 by the University of Bucharest (Romania), in 2009 by the University of Athens (Greece), and in 2019 by the University of Poznań (Poland). In 2011 he was entitled Professor Emeritus of the Ministry of Health and Social Development of Russian Federation. He is President of the International Society of Gynecological Endocrinology (ISGE), the European Society of Gynecology (ESG), and the International Academy of Human Reproduction (IAHR).

Steven R. Goldstein is Professor of Gynecology and Obstetrics at the New York University Grossman School of Medicine. Considered one of USA's top doctors in gynecology, he has published seven books on women's health topics, including menopause, perimenopause, early pregnancy monitoring, abnormal uterine bleeding, and gynecologic ultrasounds. He has also contributed numerous chapters and papers to the medical field. Dr. Goldstein is a sought-after lecturer, traveling the USA and the world to speak about issues related to obstetrics and gynecology.

Tommaso Simoncini is Professor of Obstetrics and Gynecology at the University of Pisa. He has extensively studied the mechanisms of actions of sex hormones relevant to cardiovascular disease, cancer metastasis, and brain disorders. He has published over 120 high-impact original papers. He is an officer of the International Society of Gynecological Endocrinology and European Menopause and Andropause Society and serves on the Board of the European Society of Gynecology and International Menopause Society. Prof. Simoncini is Editor of *Maturitas, Journal of Endocrinological Investigation*, and *Vascular Pharmacology*. He has received prestigious international scientific awards from the leading Societies in Obstetrics, Gynecology, and Reproductive Endocrinology.

The Use of Ultrasound in Understanding Normal and Abnormal Evaluation of the Endometrium

Steven R. Goldstein

1 Introduction

Vaginal probes for ultrasonography were introduced in the 1980s. They allow for higher frequency transducers in closer proximity to the structure being studied. This yields excellent resolution. In fact, in my first book [1], I described a concept of "sonomicroscopy" whereby we see things with the vaginal probe that one would not be able to discern with the naked eye. It is as if we were doing ultrasound through a low-power microscope. Hence, there is the ability to see structure not previously appreciated in such a non-invasive fashion.

2 The Menstrual Cycle

The endometrium consists of a basalis and a functionalis. In an idealized situation, for the 13 lunar months in a calendar year, the endometrium undergoes a cyclical journey occasionally resulting in a pregnancy, most often ending in a menses. Realize to our patients all the blood that comes out of their vagina is their "period," but to us a menses is a bleed preceded 14 days prior by ovulation.

S. R. Goldstein (✉)
New York University Grossman School of Medicine, New York University, New York, NY, USA
e-mail: steven.goldstein@nyulangone.org

A. R. Genazzani et al. (eds.), *Menstrual Bleeding and Pain Disorders from Adolescence to Menopause*, ISGE Series,
https://doi.org/10.1007/978-3-031-55300-4_1

1

3 Normal Physiology

With the onset of menses, each ovary recruits a number of follicles. These produce estradiol. The functionalis, in response to estradiol, will proliferate (Fig. 1a, b). Sonographically, this appears, ultimately, as a thickening of the endometrial echo (Fig. 2). Typically, one follicle becomes dominant leaving the other follicles behind. Prior to ovulation the endometrium will display a trilaminar, multilayered appearance (Fig. 3). After ovulation, the production of progesterone by the corpus luteum converts this estrogen primed functionalis to a secretory phase (Fig. 4b) preparing to receive a fertilized egg now traversing the fallopian tube as a zygote. When no pregnancy ensues, the endometrium breaks up and is shed as a "menses." The resulting basalis, when viewed sonographically, will appear as a thin echogenic line (Fig. 5) which represents the interface between two layers of denuded basalis (Fig. 6). There are other situations such as menopause where no estrogen is produced. The surface epithelium of the endometrium is a single layer of cuboidal cells (Fig. 7), and, when viewed sonographically, this should be a thin, white, echogenic line (Fig. 8) which, once again, is the interface of an inactive atrophic endometrium. In the situation of combination oral contraceptive pills, there is little, if any, proliferation with decidualization of what endometrium does exist, and sonographically (Fig. 9) this will appear as thin, although not quite as thin as the inactive atrophic endometrium of menopause or even the denuded basalis seen at the end of menses.

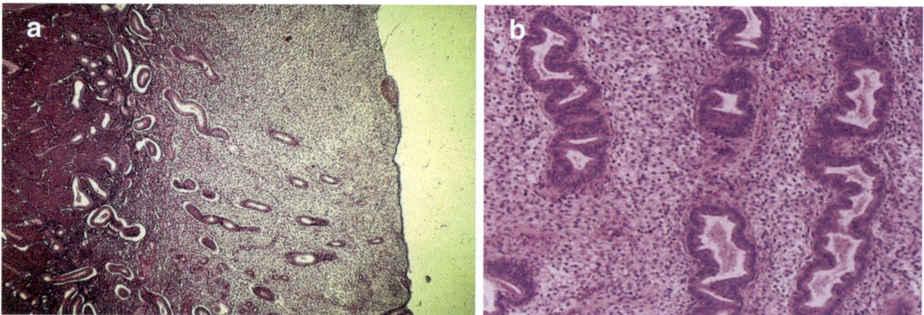

Fig. 1 (**a**) Hysterectomy specimen taken in the proliferative phase of the menstrual cycle showing proliferative endometrium. (**b**) Higher power view of proliferative endometrium showing abundant mitotic activity in virtually all of the glandular nuclei

Fig. 2 Transvaginal sonogram done in the proliferative phase of the menstrual cycle showing the beginning development of the functionalis

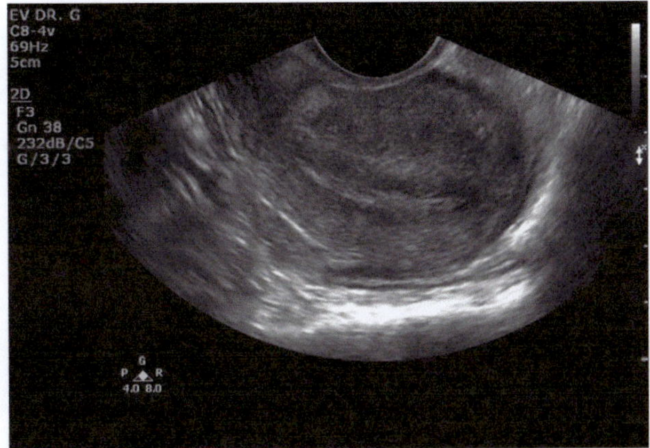

Fig. 3 Preovulatory transvaginal scan revealing a multilayered, trilaminar appearance prior to ovulation

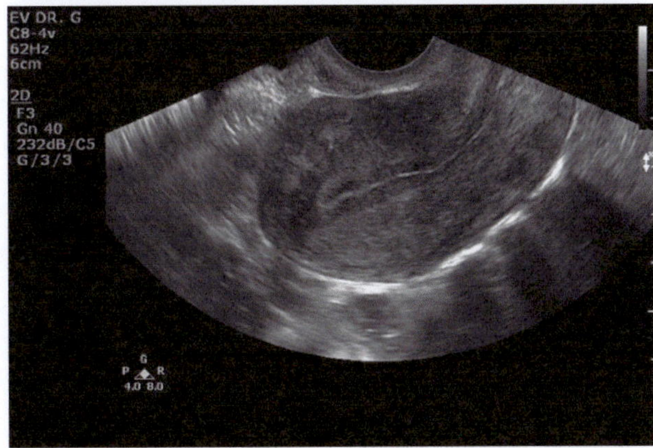

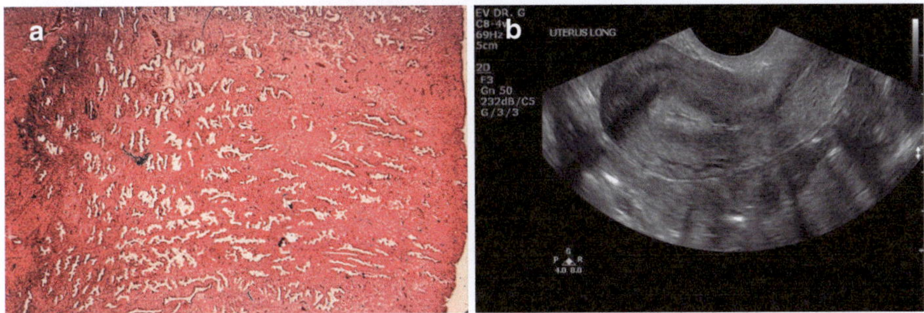

Fig. 4 (**a**) Hysterectomy specimen done in the secretory phase of the endometrium. Notice how the glands line up in a linear fashion. (**b**) Transvaginal sonogram performed in the secretory phase of the menstrual cycle in the endometrium. Under the influence of progesterone, it has become echogenic and thickened

Fig. 5 Transvaginal ultrasound done at the end of the menstrual cycle. The functionalis has been totally shed, and the remaining thin endometrial basalis, representative on ultrasound, is a thin white line representing the interface between two sides of basalis

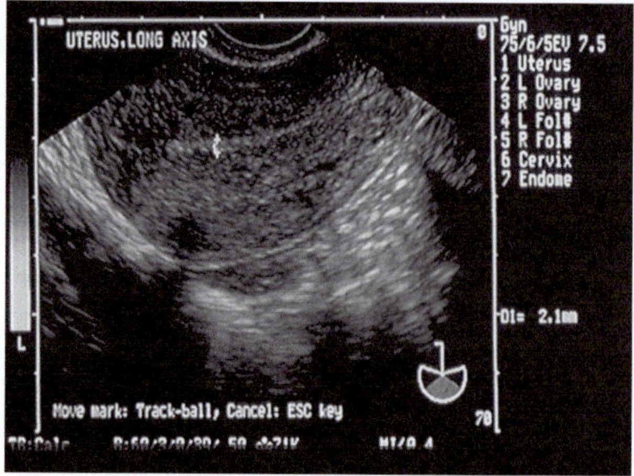

Fig. 6 Hysterectomy done in the phase of the cycle just after menstruation. The basalis remains although the functionalis has been totally sloughed

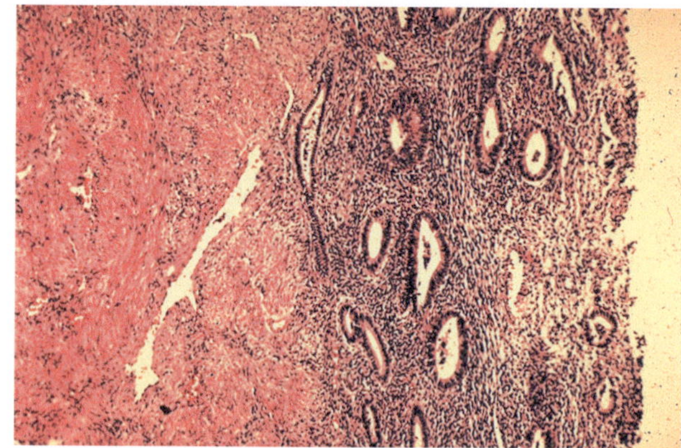

Fig. 7 Hysterectomy pathology specimen done on a menopausal patient. The surface epithelium is thin representing a single layer of low cuboidal cells

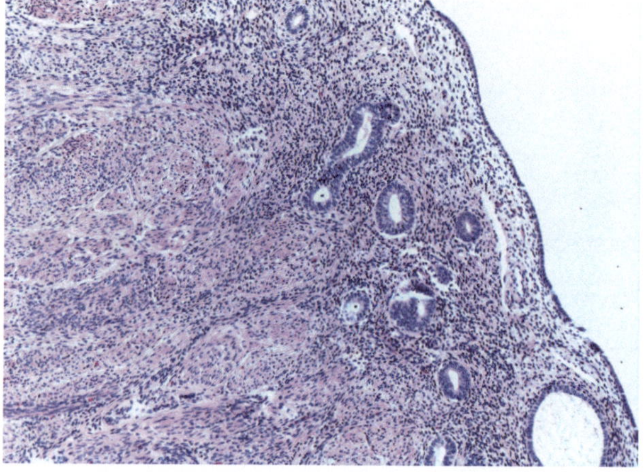

Fig. 8 Transvaginal
sonogram done on a
postmenopausal patient.
This thin, white echogenic
line represents the interface
between two layers of
inactive, atrophic
endometrium

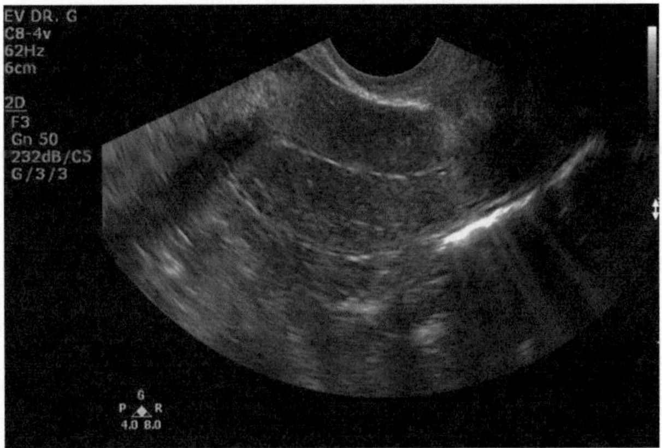

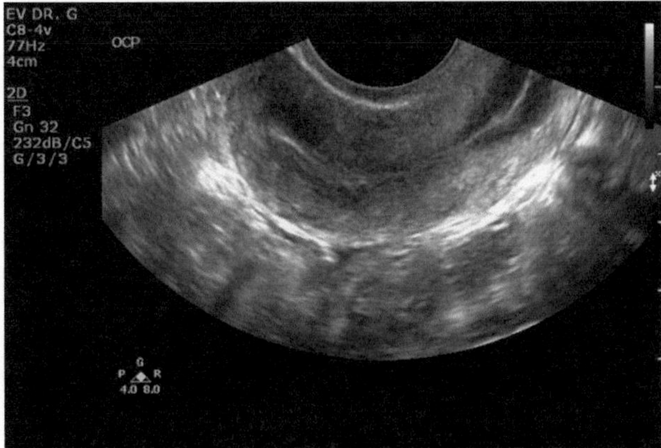

Fig. 9 Transvaginal sonogram done on a patient on birth control pills. The endometrial echo is thin (however, not as thin as a postmenstrual or postmenopausal patient). If looked at histopathologically, this would represent a decidualized layer of nonproliferative endometrium, something that does not exist in nature and is the result of the combination birth control pill

4 Pathologies of Abnormal Uterine Bleeding (AUB)

With this understanding of normal physiology and its corresponding sonographic appearance, we can explore the various causes of abnormal uterine bleeding. FIGO has introduced the PALM-COEIN system (Fig. 10). A simpler way of looking at this is structural versus non-structural reasons for AUB. The non-structural reasons will display various degrees of endometrial tissue and, thus, varying degrees of endometrial thickness. Saline infusion sonohysterography, often referred to as SIS, involves instillation of sterile saline or gel through a small catheter into the uterine cavity while performing transvaginal ultrasound. Fluid enhances sound transmission. This is well appreciated in obstetrics because the fetus is surrounded by amniotic fluid allowing wonderful resolution of fetal anatomy. In SIS, the expansion of

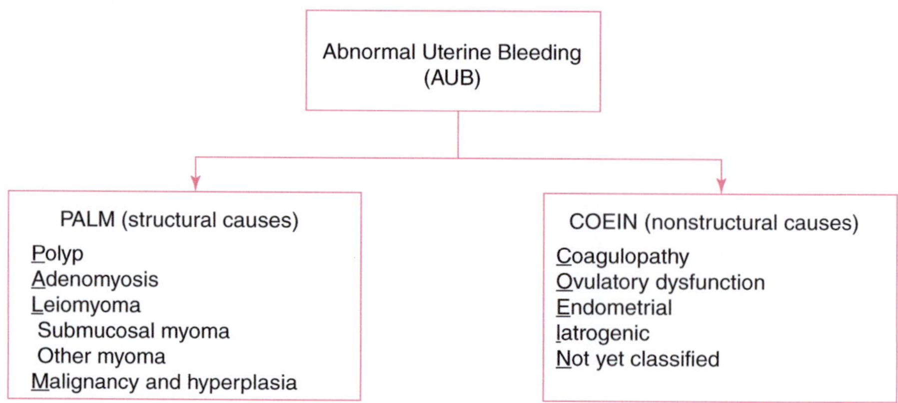

Fig. 10 PALM-COEIN nomenclature of causes of abnormal uterine bleeding

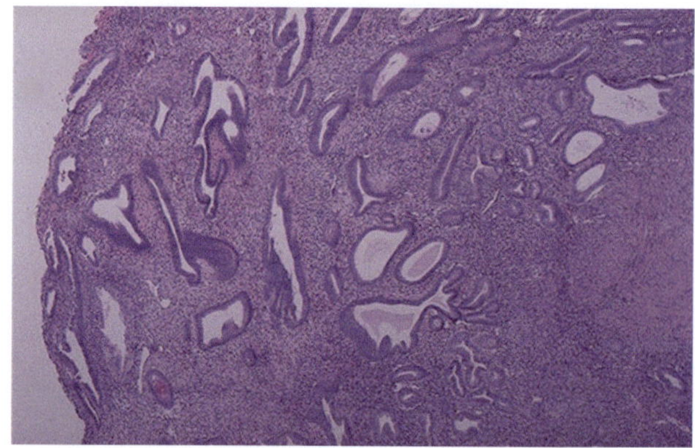

Fig. 11 Hysterectomy specimen done on a patient with simple hyperplasia. Note the abundant "back-to-back" glands arranged in a highly irregular fashion

the endometrial cavity and fluid insertion allow exquisite visualization. SIS should be thought of as a subset of transvaginal ultrasound when the endometrial echo is not sufficiently thin or is inadequately visualized for the various reasons discussed below. One study of 433 patients with perimenopausal bleeding [2] found 79% of AUB was dysfunctional anovulatory bleeding without any structural abnormality. Most of such patients, if undergoing endometrial sampling, will display proliferative endometrium and can virtually always be treated hormonally or even expectantly. Hormonal treatment is often combination oral contraceptive pills, if not contraindicated, or periodic progestogen. However, some patients will display hyperplasia (Fig. 11). Sonographically, this may be diffusely thickened on SIS (Fig. 12a, b) or focally thick (Fig. 13).

Blind endometrial sampling, although still an apparent first step to obtain histology, [3] has been shown to be less reliable if endometrial pathology occupies less

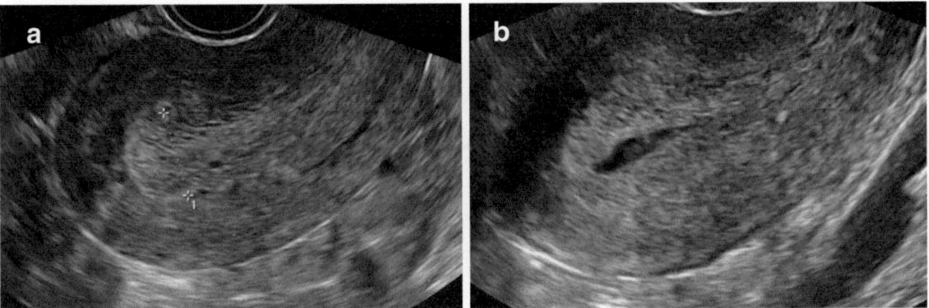

Fig. 12 (**a**) Transvaginal pelvic sonogram showing a thickened endometrial echo in a perimeno-pausal patient with abnormal uterine bleeding. (**b**) Saline infusion sonohysterogram on the patient in (**a**). This shows a symmetrically thick endometrial tissue surrounding the fluid. Endometrial sampling on this global process revealed simple hyperplasia

Fig. 13 Saline infusion sonohysterogram showing a focal area of thickness along the anterior wall, whereas the posterior wall is devoid of significant tissue. This was complex atypical hyperplasia on hysteroscopic directed sampling

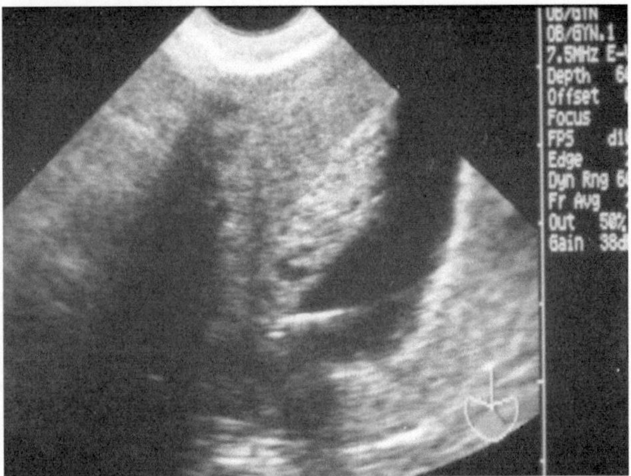

than 50% of the uterine cavity [3]. The use of saline infusion sonohysterography or newer disposable office hysteroscopes can further triage abnormal-appearing endo-metrial thickness on transvaginal ultrasound to global versus focal process. If the process is global, blind endometrial sampling remains appropriate [4]. If the process is focal, the sampling should be done under direct vision by hysteroscopy. Such cases would include focal tissue (Fig. 13), polyps (Fig. 14), or submucous myomas (Fig. 15).

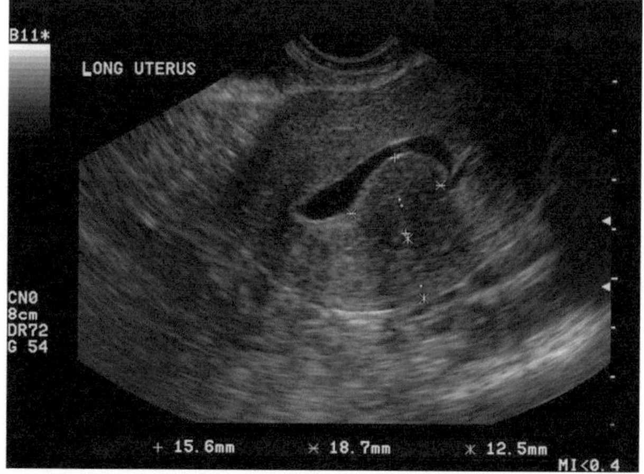

Fig. 14 Transvaginal pelvic sonogram with saline infusion sonohysterography showing an obvious polyp along the anterior wall near the fundus. This measured 2.1 cm maximum diameter. The endometrium surrounding the fluid is seen to be thin compatible with early proliferative phase of the patient. The SIS catheter can be seen along the posterior wall

Fig. 15 Transvaginal pelvic sonogram with saline infusion sonohysterogram revealing an intramural/submucosal fibroid distorting the endometrial cavity

5 Postmenopausal Bleeding

Our most junior trainees are taught that any postmenopausal bleeding is endometrial cancer until proven otherwise. Review of the literature would indicate that 1–14% of such patients will have endometrial cancer, [4] although most of these place it in the 5–10% range. The original observational studies [5–7] in postmenopausal women with bleeding consistently found that an endometrial echo on transvaginal ultrasound <5 mm was associated with lack of significant tissue. Multiple large, prospective trials, mainly out of Western Europe, caused the American College of Obstetrician and Gynecologists in 2009 [8] to opine that "when present, a thin, distinct endometrial echo on transvaginal ultrasonography 4 mm or less has a risk of malignancy of 1 in 917 and, therefore, endometrial sampling is not required." In fact, if one does a biopsy in such patients with a thin, distinct

Table 1 Endometrial thickness and incidence of cancer in postmenopausal women with bleeding

Reference	Endometrial thickness on TVUS	Number of women	Total sample of bleeding women	Number of cases of cancers	Negative predictive value
Karlson 1995[a]	$\leq$4 mm	518	1138	0	100%
Ferrazzi 1996[b]	$\leq$4 mm	336	930	2	99.4%
	$\leq$5 mm	456	930	4	99.1%
Gull 2003[c]	$\leq$4 mm	394	394	0	100%
Wong 2016[d]	$\leq$3 mm	1915	4383	5	99.7%
	$\leq$4 mm	2825	4383	10	99.6%
	$\leq$5 mm	3131	4383	11	99.6%

Expressed as a composite of above studies		
For EM $\leq$ 3 mm	5/1915 cancers	= 1 in 383
For EM $\leq$ 4 mm	12/4073 cancers	= 1 in 339
For EM $\leq$ 5 mm	15/3587 cancers	= 1 in 239

[a] Karlsson B, Granberg S, Wikland M, et al. Transvaginal ultrasonography of the endometrium in women with postmenopausal bleeding—a Nordic multicenter study. Am J Obstet Gynecol 1995;172:1488–94

[b] Ferrazzi E, Torri V, Trio D, Zannoni E, Filiberto S, Dordoni D. Sonographic endometrial thickness: a useful test to predict atrophy in patients with postmenopausal bleeding. An Italian multicenter study. Ultrasound Obstet Gynecol 1996;7:315–21

[c] Gull B, Karlsson B, Milsom I, Granberg S. Can ultrasound replace dilation and curettage? A longitudinal evaluation of postmenopausal bleeding and transvaginal sonographic measurement of the endometrium as predictors of endometrial cancer. Am J Obstet Gynecol 2003;188:401–8

[d] Wong AS, Lao TT, Cheung CW, Yeung SW, Fan HL, Ng PS, et al. Reappraisal of endometrial thickness for the detection of endometrial cancer in postmenopausal bleeding: a retrospective cohort study. BJOG 2016;123:439–46

endometrial echo on transvaginal ultrasonography, it is common to not successfully obtain tissue, or when tissue is present, it is often so scant that it is insufficient for evaluation [9, 10].

More recently, ACOG has updated its Committee Opinion [11]. It now incorporates a large Chinese study by Wong et al. [12] and gives a risk of endometrial cancer for endometrial thicknesses of 3, 4, and 5 mm, respectively (Table 1). However, it still states that for average-risk women, a cutoff of $\leq$4 mm is still appropriate.

6 Limitations of Transvaginal Ultrasound

Transvaginal ultrasound has some significant limitations. It is a technical procedure that does not always reveal meaningful results. Not all uteri will lend themselves to produce a reliable endometrial echo. Previous surgery, coexisting leiomyomas, axial orientation, marked obesity, and adenomyosis can all result in an inability to find a reliable endometrial echo. As discussed above, in such cases fluid enhancement by saline infusion sonohysterography will easily highlight the endometrial cavity in a simple, painless office procedure. SIS will allow differentiation to (1) no anatomic pathology (no biopsy necessary), (2) globally thick endometrium (blind sampling appropriate), and (3) focal abnormalities that should be done under direct vision.

In that study of 433 perimenopausal women [2], 44 (10.2%) had SIS because of inability to adequately visualize an endometrial echo. These were perimenopausal women studied because of AUB. A recent study [13] of 472 consecutive asymptomatic postmenopausal women found that in 38.1% an endometrial echo adequate for appropriate measurement for diagnostic purposes could not be identified. Of the overall cohort, the reasons for nonvisualization were fibroids (20.1%), axial uterine orientation (10.6%), and adenomyosis (7.4%). These women were, on average, 14.1 years past menopause. There was no difference in the ability to visualize an endometrial echo based on years since menopause, but mean BMI was significantly greater in the nonvisualized cohort (mean BMI 25.4) versus the visualized group (mean BMI 23.9, $p = 0.015$). In the study by Wong [12], the nonvisualization rate was 20.2%. However, these were postmenopausal women with bleeding and averaged 5 years since menopause.

Another limitation of transvaginal ultrasound in premenopausal women underscores the importance of where in the bleeding cycle an ultrasound is performed. Ideally, transvaginal ultrasound is done in patients who are cycling as soon as possible after the bleeding ends when the endometrium is expected to be as thin as it will be all month long. The uterus is a rugged organ. Many women have had pregnancies, miscarriages, cesarean sections, myomectomies, etc. As tissue proliferates, it is not always topographically homogeneous. Examination later in the cycle, either with sonohysterography or hysteroscopy, can reveal very irregular surface of the endometrium which is sometimes referred to as endometrial moguls (Fig. 16) and should not be mistaken for pathology. In such patients, liberal use of a progestogen

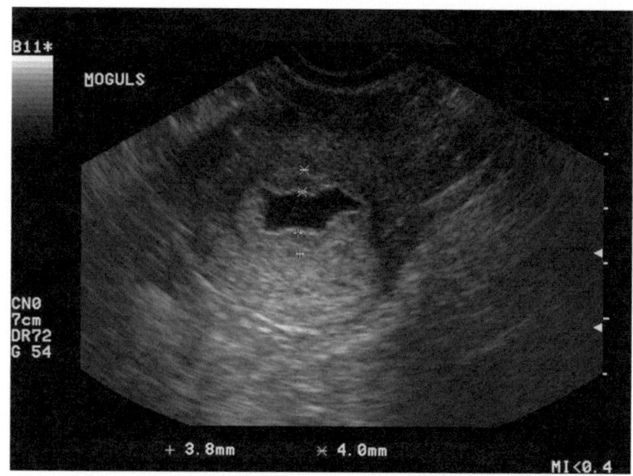

Fig. 16 Transvaginal pelvic sonogram done in the luteal phase of the menstrual cycle. The endometrium is thickened; however, it is heterogeneous irregular in its topography. Such an appearance has been labeled as endometrial "moguls" indicative of the fact that as the functionalis proliferates and then thickens in the secretory phase, it is not always topographically homogeneous

challenge test as well as appropriate timing of the ultrasound examination after withdrawal bleed is crucial.

7   Summary

The use of high-frequency transvaginal ultrasound probes and the occasional need for fluid enhancement with saline infusion have allowed us easy access for visualization of normal and abnormal findings in the endometrial cavity. Understanding its utility as well as its limitations will improve the ability of healthcare providers to deliver optimal care to patients.

References

1. Goldstein S. Endovaginal ultrasound. 1st ed. New York: Alan R. Liss Co.; 1988.
2. Goldstein S, Zeltser I, Horan C. Ultrasonography-based triage for perimenopausal patients with abnormal uterine bleeding. Am J Obstet Gynecol. 1997;177:102–8.
3. American College of Obstetricians and Gynecologists. Committee Opinion No. 128: diagnosis of abnormal uterine bleeding in reproductive age women. Obstet Gynecol. 2012;120:197–206.
4. Goldstein S. Modern evaluation of the endometrium. Obstet Gynecol. 2010;116:168–76.
5. Goldstein S, Nachtigall M, Snyder J. Endometrial assessment by vaginal ultrasonography before endometrial sampling in patients with postmenopausal bleeding. Am J Obstet Gynecol. 1990;163:119–23.
6. Varner R, Sparks J, Cameron C. Transvaginal sonography of the endometrium in postmenopausal women. Obstet Gynecol. 1991;78:195–9.
7. Granberg S, Wikland M, Karlsson B. Endometrial thickness as measured by endovaginal ultrasonography for identifying endometrial abnormality. Am J Obstet Gynecol. 1991;164:47–52.
8. American College of Obstetricians and Gynecologists. Committee Opinion No. 426: The role of transvaginal ultrasonography in the evaluation of postmenopausal bleeding. Obstet Gynecol. 2009;113:462–4.
9. Elsandabesee D, Greenwood P. The performance of Pipelle endometrial sampling in a dedicated postmenopausal bleeding clinic. J Obstet Gynaecol. 2005;25:32–4.
10. Dijkhuizen F, Mol B, Brolmann H. The accuracy of endometrial sampling in the diagnosis of patients with endometrial carcinoma and hyperplasia: a meta-analysis. Cancer. 2000;89:1765–72.
11. American College of Obstetricians and Gynecologists. Committee Opinion No. 734: the role of transvaginal ultrasonography in evaluating the endometrium of women with postmenopausal bleeding. Obstet Gynecol. 2018;131:e124–9.
12. Wong A, Lao T, Cheung C. Reappraisal of endometrial thickness for the detection of endometrial cancer in postmenopausal bleeding: a retrospective cohort study. BJOG. 2016;123:439–46.
13. Goldstein SR, Khafaga A. Ability to successfully image the endometrial echo on transvaginal ultrasound in asymptomatic postmenopausal women. Ultrasound Obstet Gynecol. 2021;58:625–9.

Sex Steroid Hormones in the Treatment of Menstrual Cycle Disorders

Ardito Marisa, A. Giannini, T. Fidecicchi, Tommaso Simoncini, and Andrea R. Genazzani

1   Introduction

As is well known, the primary use of sex steroid hormones is due to their contraceptive effect. However, they may be exploited for therapeutic purposes in different clinical conditions with satisfying extra-contraceptive benefits. Therapeutic effects can be achieved by ovulation inhibition, antiestrogenic, antiandrogenic, and progestin effects. Some of the positive effects induced by progestins are enhanced by the estrogen component, e.g., the antiandrogenic effect of some progestins is enhanced with higher doses of EE, e.g., the 30 µg. However, reduction in the dosage of the estrogen component has made estrogen-progestin therapies more tolerable to patients by reducing not only side effects but also the impact on liver metabolism and thromboembolic risk [1]. Hormonal therapy with estrogen-progestin represents one of the most essential and versatile treatments with immediate benefits on women's problems such as seborrhea, dysmenorrhea, acne, and hirsutism. Long-term benefits are also relevant, particularly of protection from several malignancies, foremost among them ovarian cancer. Many menstrual cycle disorders gain benefit from estrogen-progestin therapy, particularly dysmenorrhea, endometriosis, anovulation, PCOS, abnormal uterine bleeding, etc. After an accurate medical history, it has long been clear that the prescription of these treatments is accompanied by few risks for women compared with the benefits.

A. Marisa · A. Giannini (✉) · T. Fidecicchi · T. Simoncini · A. R. Genazzani
Division of Obstetrics and Gynecology, Department of Clinical and Experimental Medicine, University of Pisa, Pisa, Italy
e-mail: andrea.giannini@unipi.it; t.fidecicchi@gmail.co; tommaso.simoncini@unipi.it

A. R. Genazzani et al. (eds.), *Menstrual Bleeding and Pain Disorders from Adolescence to Menopause*, ISGE Series,
https://doi.org/10.1007/978-3-031-55300-4_2

2 Dysmenorrhea

The prevalence of dysmenorrhea is between 16% and 91% in women of reproductive age, with debilitating pain observed in 2–29% [2]. Agarwal et al. showed the prevalence of dysmenorrhea to be 80% in adolescents, and approximately 40% had severe dysmenorrhea [3]. Dysmenorrhea is classified into primary and secondary. Primary is prevalent in adolescence and is characterized by cramp-like pain, often disabling, that occurs during menstruation without underlying pathology. The symptoms associated with dysmenorrhea include gastrointestinal symptoms such as nausea, bloating, diarrhea, constipation, vomiting, and indigestion. Also, irritability, headache, and low back pain are prevalent among women with primary dysmenorrhea. Tiredness and dizziness are also associated with dysmenorrhea. The secondary form has the same clinical features as the primary, but there sometimes is a headline disorder or disease at its base, such as adenomyosis, endometriosis, pelvic inflammatory disease, pelvic adhesions, intrauterine devices, or ovarian cysts. The first-line therapy is represented by classic pain relievers such as nonsteroidal anti-inflammatory drugs, which can induce pain relief in about 70–90% of patients, compared with placebo [4–6] both when taken alone or in combination with hormonal contraceptives [7]. In cases of primary dysmenorrhea resistant to treatment as a second line of treatment approach, in case of non-response or non-tolerance to different analgesics, it may be appropriate to start treatment with hormonal contraceptive therapy (COC). COC can also be offered as first-line therapy in sexually active patients, preventing dysmenorrhea and pregnancy by combining estrogen and progesterone [8]. Hormonal contraceptives act by preventing menstrual pain, suppressing ovulation, thinning the endometrial rhyme, decreasing endometrial prostaglandin levels and the frequency of myometrial contractions, and reducing the magnitude of menstrual flow when taken for several months in a row. Randomized studies in fertile women treated with hormonal therapy show moderate efficacy in pain relief [9, 10]. A meta-analysis of studies reported a therapeutic benefit compared with a placebo and a similar result for both pills with estrogen doses ≤35 µg and doses >35 µg [10]. In addition, lower-dose formulations such as 20 µg ethinyl estradiol also appear to be effective in reducing pain [11–13]. The beneficial effects of low-dose estrogen COCs have long been known, but it is necessary to consider a woman's age before prescribing in order to assess the impact on bone mass. In mature, premenopausal women, COCs have been shown to have no or a beneficial effect on skeletal health, as assessed by both BMD and fracture rates [14]. Other studies have examined whether the skeletal effects vary by dose of ethinylestradiol (15 vs. 20 µg) [15] or by different progestins (drospirenone or gestodene) [16]. In both cases, change in spine BMD did not differ between COC users and controls. However, other studies indicate that COC use in adolescence can have a negative effect on bone mineral acquisition, especially in the first 3 years post menarche. Researchers found lower rates of bone mineral accrual in adolescents using low-dose (20 µg ethinyl estradiol) COC formulations compared with controls not using hormonal contraceptives [17, 18]. Some progestins, for example, COCs containing

CMA (chlormadinone acetate), can induce improvement or remission of symptoms due to the ability of this progestin to directly suppress cyclo-oxygenase. COCs with drospirenone, which is characterized by a potent antimineralocorticoid effect, especially with the 24/4 regimen, has been recognized by the FDA as the most suitable treatment for premenstrual dysphoric disorder (PMDD) [19, 20]. Other studies have focused instead on the type of regimen used, recording a decrease of menstrual symptoms with prolonged or continuous administration compared with cyclic dosing [21, 22]. However, for patients in whom conventional cyclic dosing (21 days of drug/7 days of placebo) of an oral contraceptive formulation does not provide sufficient relief of dysmenorrhea, it is reasonable to switch to a formulation with a reduced hormonal interval (e.g., a 24/4 formulation) or to an extended-cycle formulation. Other hormonal contraceptives that treat dysmenorrhea include transdermal patches or the vaginal ring, injectable or implantable contraceptives, or levonorgestrel-releasing intrauterine devices. A review of 12 randomized trials comparing the vaginal ring with the pill concluded that both methods reduce dysmenorrhea [23]. In contrast, a randomized trial of COCs shows that dysmenorrhea is slightly more common among women who use the patch versus pills [24]. Another effective treatment can be progestin-only products since they induce endometrial atrophy, reducing dysmenorrhea. Although they have some more common side effects than combined contraceptives, such as irregular bleeding, the advantage of progestin-only compounds is that they can be used safely where a contraceptive with estrogen is contraindicated. However, some of these methods do not inhibit ovulation as effectively as estrogen-progestin therapy, thus reducing the contraceptive effect. A progestin that is effective in reducing dysmenorrhea is the levonorgestrel-releasing intrauterine device (LNG-IUD), also due to the amenorrhea rate of about 20% after 1 year of use [25–27]. In contrast, patients with copper T380A IUD devices experience often increased dysmenorrhea. In a large 3-year clinical trial evaluating the safety and efficacy of the subcutaneous etonogestrel implant, more than three-quarters of participants who had been complaining of primary dysmenorrhea reported improvement at the end of treatment [28]. Improvement has been shown in dysmenorrhea, non-menstrual pelvic pain, and dyspareunia, especially in women with histologically documented endometriosis [29].

3 Endometriosis/Adenomyosis

Patients with endometriosis suffer from painful periods, pain with intercourse, pain with bowel movements, excessive bleeding, and infertility. Treatment options include nonsteroidal analgesics, hormonal contraceptives, gonadotropin-releasing hormone (GnRH) analogues and antagonists, and aromatase inhibitors. The choice depends on the severity of symptoms, side effects of the drugs, treatment efficacy, contraceptive needs, cost, and availability [30]. Whatever therapy is chosen, this does not increase fertility rates, decrease the number or size of endometriomas, or even treat complications of deep endometriosis such as ureteral obstruction [31, 32].

The medical treatment of endometriosis is based on the concept that sex hormones modulate ectopic endometrial tissue. The therapeutic strategy is to create a hypoestrogenic hormonal climate designed to reduce the tropism of endometriotic lesions. Combined estrogen-progestin contraceptives are the first-line treatment for most women with endometriosis-related pain because they can be taken long-term, are well tolerated, and are easy to use, plus they provide additional benefits [33]. All these effects result from hormone therapy-induced suppression of ovarian function, suppression of endometriotic implant growth, and, consequently, pain [34]. The underlying therapeutic mechanism is the decidualization and subsequent atrophy of the endometrial glands [35]. It is generally appropriate to start with a continuous COC containing 20 mcg of ethinylestradiol [36] depending on the patient's age. Although both cyclic and continuous hormonal regimens effectively reduce endometriosis-related pain [37], two systematic reviews have reported that continuous COC regimens would be more valuable in treating secondary dysmenorrhea than cyclic regimens [38]. However, in conditions where estrogen is contraindicated, progestin-only therapy (an intrauterine device with levonorgestrel, contraceptive implant, or pill) can halt menstrual periods and the growth of endometrial implants and thus can be considered an alternative treatment option. Furthermore, compared with danazol, progestins are better tolerated, have no androgenic side effects, and have a less detrimental impact on the lipid profile. The most frequently used progestins include medroxyprogesterone acetate or 19-nortestosterone derivatives, norethindrone acetate, and dienogest [39]. Specifically, MPA can be administered as an intramuscular or subcutaneous injection every 3 months. In contrast, dienogest can be prescribed as an oral pill or combined with estradiol valerate as part of a multiphasic oral contraceptive pill. Side effects of progestin treatment can be irregular uterine bleeding, amenorrhea, weight gain, and mood changes. Alternative options for progestins in the treatment include ethylnorgestrienone (a synthetic steroid), the subcutaneous implant etonogestrel, and the intrauterine device levonorgestrel. Some observational studies show that the subcutaneous implant effectively decreases the intensity of endometriosis-related pain (dyspareunia, dysmenorrhea, non-menstrual pelvic pain) [40]. LNG-IUD has been shown to result in decreased endometrial proliferation and increased apoptosis in the glandular and endometrial stroma [41]. Reference guidelines of the Royal College of Obstetricians and Gynecologists state that through the use of this medicated intrauterine device, pain is reduced for at least 3 years. LNG-IUD is also indicated to induce a down-regulation of estrogen receptors in the glandular and stromal compartments of endometrial tissues, preventing further stimulation by estrogen and leading to atrophy and shrinkage of endometriotic foci [42]. A review of three studies concluded that postoperative use of LNG-IUD reduces the recurrence of dysmenorrhea in women with surgically confirmed endometriosis [43–45].

4 Polycystic Ovary Syndrome (PCOS)

Many women of childbearing age suffer from oligomenorrhea and PCOS, a disorder associated with chronic anovulation and hyperandrogenism. Management of clinical manifestations of PCOS includes lifestyle changes and combined hormonal contraceptives (COCs). Estrogen reaches antiandrogenic properties by influencing the hepatic synthesis of sex hormone-binding globulin (SHBG) and reducing the free testosterone that can bind the androgen receptor [46].This antiandrogen effect is more prominent with the use of EE than with the use of natural estrogen [46]. A systematic review of 42 experimental studies with meta-analysis demonstrated that independent of the type of progestogens present in combined oral contraceptives (COCs) containing 20–35 μg EE, the use of COCs was associated with a 61% reduction of free testosterone levels [47]. Moreover, the progestogen suppresses luteinizing hormone secretion and blocks ovulation and androgen production. Therefore, the effect will be the control of the menstrual cycle and the reduction of some clinical signs, such as acne, seborrhea and hirsutism, changes in mood and behavior, anxiety, and depression. Due to its antiandrogenic action, the progestin compound must be selected judiciously. There are currently four progestins with specific antiandrogenic activity: cyproterone acetate, dienogest, drospirenone, and chlormadinone acetate. Cyproterone acetate is the progestin with the highest antiandrogenic activity, although it induces a relatively higher rate of side effects, including headaches [1]. PCOS is associated with clinical and metabolic comorbidities that may limit the prescription of COCs in women with PCOS. Systemic arterial hypertension, obesity, dyslipidemia, metabolic syndrome, and type 2 diabetes mellitus (DM2) can coexist with menstrual problems in women with PCOS [48, 49]. Progestogen-only contraceptives (POCs) are typically considered a safer option for women presenting with cardiovascular comorbidities and so in cases of contraindications to COC.

5 Hyperandrogenic Disorders

All COCs can antagonize hyperandrogenism by the effect on gonadotropin secretion and by the effect of estrogens on hepatic sex hormone-binding globulin (SHBG) synthesis, reducing the share of free androgens and a reduction of their negative action at the level of sebaceous glands, hair follicles, and scalp. The antiandrogenic effect of oral contraceptives can be traced back to the progestin component, particularly COCs containing third-generation progestins; some molecules such as cyproterone acetate, dienogest, drospirenone, and chlormadinone acetate, which act by blocking androgen receptors and inhibiting the action of circulating androgens, are preferable. The progestin with the greatest antiandrogenic effect is cyproterone acetate. In addition to improving the signs and symptoms of hyperandrogenism, these oral contraceptives lead to a normalization of ovarian structure and ovarian volume in women with PCOS, with a numerical reduction of follicles [50, 51]. Even after discontinuation of contraceptive therapies, these structural changes typically persist 4–6 months at least. Aggregate analysis of two randomized placebo-controlled trials with a total of 893 women with moderate facial acne found that patients treated with ethinylestradiol 20 µg/drospirenone 3 mg for six cycles were more likely to achieve skin improvement than those treated with placebo [52]. The study by Palombo-Kinne et al. also confirms the superiority in terms of efficacy of the oral contraceptive containing ethinylestradiol 30 µg/dienogest 2 mg over placebo [53]. The efficacy of contraceptive preparations on the signs of hyperandrogenism (acne, hirsutism, seborrhea, and alopecia) is time-dependent; therefore, in such a case, whatever contraceptive pill is administered, the minimum period of treatment should be 4–5 months, possibly up to 12 months. In addition, using the contraceptive pill for long periods protects the patient from the recurrence of hyperandrogenism and associated conditions, including chronic anovulation and infertility [54]. Oral contraceptives can be used alone or with other medications to approach both acne and hirsutism. In addition to basal hormone therapy, some studies have shown efficacy in combination with spironolactone [55, 56]. When choosing the right therapy and type of progestin, it's important to consider some precautions. For example, drospirenone is known to have potential potassium-sparing effects due to its anti-mineralocorticoid activity. However, it has been shown that healthy women taking COCs with drospirenone are no more likely to develop hyperkalemia than women taking other COCs with other types of progestins [57, 58]. Package labeling recommends potassium monitoring during the first month for women taking additional medications that predispose to hyperkalemia (e.g., spironolactone, nonsteroidal anti-inflammatory drugs [NSAIDs], angiotensin-converting enzyme inhibitors) [59].

During childbearing, women with PCOS are more likely to have severe symptoms related to behavior, mood, sleep, and metabolism, particularly insulin resistance and compensatory hyperinsulinemia. Therefore, hormone replacement therapy is crucial in maintaining an adequate steroid balance [60].

6 Oncologic Risk

Established epidemiological data show that hormonal contraception has an overall effect in reducing cancer occurrence [61]. A 44-year observational study, involving a total of 388,505 women per year, reported exciting data about the reduction of cancer incidence in women using hormonal contraceptives compared with non-users [62]. In particular, the cancers mainly affected in a positive sense by long-term hormonal contraceptive use were found to be colorectal, endometrial, ovarian, lymphatic, and hematopoietic cancers. Moreover, the reduction in the incidence of endometrial, ovarian, and colorectal cancer persists for at least 30 years after COC discontinuation. Regarding endometrial cancer, the protective effect of estrogen-progestin, progestin-only, or intrauterine appears to be time therapy-related and persists after discontinuation [63]. The positive effect is based on the antiproliferative effect on the endometrium, which reduces the risk of endometrial hyperplasia and cancer. The reduction in the risk of both malignant and borderline ovarian epithelial carcinoma, but not mucinous epithelial carcinoma, is proportional to the duration of hormonal contraceptive use and persists for more than 30 years [64]. The most significant effect is the use of oral estrogen-progestins, which inhibit ovulation, suppress gonadotropin secretion, and reduce retrograde menstruation. However, prolonged use of LNG-IUD has also shown a protective effect on this type of cancer [65].

7   Abnormal Uterine Bleeding

Abnormal uterine bleeding is one of the most common gynecologic disorders in patients of childbearing age, characterized by bleeding occurring between the menstrual cycle and the next in the absence of hormone therapy. In a minority of cases, the cause can be traced to systemic and neoplastic diseases, drug intake, sudden weight loss, and intense physical activity. In most cases, it is due to the immaturity of the hypothalamic-pituitary-ovarian axis that characterizes the first 2 years after menarche or its decay during the perimenopausal period, leading to anovulatory production of sex steroids. Women may experience abnormal bleeding due to ovulatory deficits. Anovulation means no efficient progesterone production, thus inducing an abnormal control of endometrium and its potential hyperplastic evolution. Consequent bleeding occurs when the endometrium proliferates beyond the ability of endogenous estrogen to maintain its integrity. Therefore, administering exogenous estrogen or progestin by allowing further cell proliferation stabilizes the endometrial rhyme with a hemostatic effect [66]. Therefore, first-line therapy combined with oral estrogen-progestin therapy is useful, in combination or not, with hemostatic agents, for patients with anovulatory uterine bleeding. In patients with severe anovulatory bleeding associated with anemia, the initial choice should be a monophasic combined oral contraceptive pill with estrogen (e.g., 35 or 50 µg ethinylestradiol) combined with 0.5 mg of norgestrel or 1 mg of norethindrone administered every 4–6 h until the bleeding resolves, subsequently scaling the dose to one tablet every 8 h for 3 days, then one every 12 h for up to 2 weeks, and finally one pill once daily [67]. During this time, the patient must discard the placebo pills, reintroducing them only upon complete resolution of the bleeding and of the anemia. Oral progestin-only therapy is an option if there are contraindications to estrogen use (e.g., migraine with aura, arterial or venous thromboembolic disease, liver disease) [68, 69]. Among the various progestin-only oral formulations, norethindrone 5–10 mg is a viable option when administered up to four times daily depending on the severity of the patient's bleeding, subsequently scaling the dose according to appropriate therapeutic schedules once resolution of symptoms is achieved. The most widely used schedule involves taking norethindrone twice daily for 7 days, followed by once daily until the start of maintenance therapy [70]. After the

Table 1 Use of hormonal therapies for the treatment of menstrual cycle disorders

Pathological profile	Therapeutic approach
Endometriosis/dysmenorrhea	Chlormadinone acetate Dienogest LNG-IUD Continuous regime > standard
PMS (premenstrual syndrome)	CO with drospirenone or Chlormadinone Natural estrogen > ethinylestradiol, EE Regime esteso o continuativo
PCOS, hyperandrogenism	EE > natural estrogen Cyproterone acetate Dienogest Drospirenone
Drop in sexual desire	Natural estrogen (17 beta estradiol)
AUB (abnormal uterine bleeding)	Medroxyprogesterone acetate depot (DMPA) LNG-IUD

resolution of the acute episode, oral combination regimens are the most used for maintenance; either a cyclic or extended or continuous regimen may be chosen. For example, in clinical trials in women with regular menstrual flow, it is observed that extended-cycle COC formulations in which placebo tablets are replaced by low-dose ethinyl estradiol appear to reduce unplanned bleeding [71]. For patients who desire contraception but show contraindications to estrogen use, progestin-only oral therapy (norethindrone, micronized progesterone, or medroxyprogesterone), levonorgestrel-releasing intrauterine device, subcutaneous implantation, and depo-medroxyprogesterone acetate (DMPA) can also be used. Medroxyprogesterone acetate depot (DMPA) is administered by intramuscular or subcutaneous injection at 90-day intervals; it inhibits ovulation, eliminating uterine bleeding, in about 50–75% of patients. DMPA is preferred to induce amenorrhea where estrogen-progestin contraceptives or the intrauterine device is contraindicated.

LNG-IUD, for example, is a highly effective and easy-to-use treatment option, being able to be proposed as a first-line option for the treatment of uterine bleeding in women who do not desire pregnancy and providing protection against hyperplasia and endometrial cancer.

The use of hormonal therapies in the treatment of menstrual cycle disorders is summarized in Table 1.

8 New Trends

Not only estrogen but also androgens contribute to the maintenance of tropism and function of the sexual sphere and female genitalia [72]. In addition, the role of androgens is crucial in all phases of the sexual response, particularly in the stimulation of desire. Research and clinical evidence support a positive effect of testosterone therapy on sexual desire when premenopausal physiologic levels are maintained

[73]. Androgen restored contraception (ARC) is a recent form of oral contraception with the aim to preserve sexual function and prevent mood disturbances. This is achieved by adding dehydroepiandrosterone (DHEA) to the COC. Dehydroepiandrosterone (DHEA) is an inactive steroid precursor that is converted to estrogen and androgen vaginally [72]. Taking COCs reduces total and free testosterone levels and increases SHBG concentrations. Coelingh Bennink H. J. T. et al. showed how, with the addition of 50 mg of DHEA, normal levels of testosterone are maintained or restored during the use of a contraceptive pill [74]. By coadministration with DHEA, physiological levels of total and free testosterone are restored while using EE/LNG. With EE/DRSP, only the free testosterone level is normalized by DHEA coadministration. In another randomized, double-blind, placebo-controlled study, van Lunsen R. H. W. et al. showed how maintaining or restoring physiological testosterone concentrations by the coadministration of DHEA to the COC may prevent negative effects on sexuality, especially in women with free testosterone levels in the highest physiological range during DHEA coadministration [75].

Even though health benefits and therapeutic uses of oral contraceptives were identified more than 10 years ago, women today are largely unaware of these, and they tend to overestimate their risk.

In the last 2 years, a new contraceptive therapy using estrogen E4, estetrol, has been introduced. Its safety profile in multiple areas could help adherence to this therapy. Preclinical studies have largely demonstrated that the combination of E4 with drospirenone (DSP), one of the progestins of least biological impact, is optimal [76]. It has been showed that the E4/DSP combination (15 mg/3 mg) has minimal impact on hemostasis, coagulation factors, fibrinolysis, angiotensinogen, cholesterol, and triglycerides [76, 77] with optimal endometrial control also compared with the E4/levonorgestrel combination [78]. In fact, the characteristics of E4 are thus such that it enhances the effects of EE and E2 itself while maintaining contraceptive efficacy. We are therefore close to an evolution in hormonal therapies, and because of this counseling and education are necessary to help women make well-informed health-care decisions and improve compliance.

References

1. Schindler AE. Non-contraceptive benefits of oral hormonal contraceptives. Int J Endocrinol Metab. 2012;11(1):41–7.
2. Ju H, Jones M, Mishra G. The prevalence and risk factors of dysmenorrhea. Epidemiol Rev. 2014;36:104–13.
3. Agarwal K, Agarwal A. A study of dysmenorrhea during menstruation in adolescent girls. Indian J Community Med. 2010;35:159.
4. Zhang WY, Li Wan Po A. Efficacy of minor analgesics in primary dysmenorrhoea: a systematic review. BJOG Int J Obstet Gynaecol. 1998;105:780–9.
5. French L. Dysmenorrhea. Am Fam Physician. 2005;71:285–91.

6. Marjoribanks J, Proctor M, Farquhar C, Derks RS. Nonsteroidal anti-inflammatory drugs for dysmenorrhoea. Cochrane Database Syst Rev. 2010;(1):CD001751. https://doi.org/10.1002/14651858.CD001751.pub2.
7. Chan WY, Yusoff Dawood M, Fuchs F. Prostaglandins in primary dysmenorrhea. Am J Med. 1981;70:535–41.
8. ACOG Committee Opinion No. 760. Summary: dysmenorrhea and endometriosis in the adolescent. Obstet Gynecol. 2018;132:1517–8.
9. Davis AR, Westhoff C, O'Connell K, Gallagher N. Oral contraceptives for dysmenorrhea in adolescent girls: a randomized trial. Obstet Gynecol. 2005;106:97–104.
10. Wong CL, Farquhar C, Roberts H, Proctor M. Oral contraceptive pill for primary dysmenorrhoea. Cochrane Database Syst Rev. 2009(4):CD002120. https://doi.org/10.1002/14651858.CD002120.pub3.
11. Petraglia F, Parke S, Serrani M, Mellinger U, Römer T. Estradiol valerate plus dienogest versus ethinylestradiol plus levonorgestrel for the treatment of primary dysmenorrhea. Int J Gynecol Obstet. 2014;125:270–4.
12. Callejo J, Díaz J, Ruiz A, García RM. Effect of a low-dose oral contraceptive containing 20 µg ethinylestradiol and 150 µg desogestrel on dysmenorrhea. Contraception. 2003;68:183–8.
13. Hendrix SL, Alexander NJ. Primary dysmenorrhea treatment with a desogestrel-containing low-dose oral contraceptive. Contraception. 2002;66:393–9.
14. Nappi C, Bifulco G, Tommaselli GA, Gargano V, Di Carlo C. Hormonal contraception and bone metabolism: a systematic review. Contraception. 2012;86:606–21.
15. Nappi C, et al. Effects of a low-dose and ultra-low-dose combined oral contraceptive use on bone turnover and bone mineral density in young fertile women: a prospective controlled randomized study. Contraception. 2003;67:355–9.
16. Nappi C, et al. Effects of an oral contraceptive containing drospirenone on bone turnover and bone mineral density. Obstet Gynecol. 2005;105:53–60.
17. Cromer BA, et al. Depot medroxyprogesterone acetate, oral contraceptives and bone mineral density in a cohort of adolescent girls. J Adolesc Health. 2004;35:434–41.
18. Brajic TS, et al. Combined hormonal contraceptives use and bone mineral density changes in adolescent and young women in a prospective population-based Canada-wide observational study. J Musculoskelet Neuronal Interact. 2018;18:227–36.
19. Huber JC, Bentz E-K, Ott J, Tempfer CB. Non-contraceptive benefits of oral contraceptives. Expert Opin Pharmacother. 2008;9:2317–25.
20. Sillem M. Yasminelle®: a new low-dose combined oral contraceptive containing drospirenone. Womens Health. 2006;2:551–9.
21. Edelman A, Gallo MF, Jensen JT, Nichols MD, Grimes DA. Continuous or extended cycle vs. cyclic use of combined hormonal contraceptives for contraception. Cochrane Database Syst Rev. 2005;(3):CD004695. https://doi.org/10.1002/14651858.CD004695.pub2.
22. Machado RB, de Melo NR, Maia H. Bleeding patterns and menstrual-related symptoms with the continuous use of a contraceptive combination of ethinylestradiol and drospirenone: a randomized study. Contraception. 2010;81:215–22.
23. Roumen FJME. The contraceptive vaginal ring compared with the combined oral contraceptive pill: a comprehensive review of randomized controlled trials. Contraception. 2007;75:420–9.
24. Audet M-C. Evaluation of contraceptive efficacy and cycle control of a transdermal contraceptive patch vs an oral contraceptive: a randomized controlled trial. JAMA. 2001;285:2347.
25. Varma R, Sinha D, Gupta JK. Non-contraceptive uses of levonorgestrel-releasing hormone system (LNG-IUS)—a systematic enquiry and overview. Eur J Obstet Gynecol Reprod Biol. 2006;125:9–28.
26. Lindh I, Milsom I. The influence of intrauterine contraception on the prevalence and severity of dysmenorrhea: a longitudinal population study. Hum Reprod. 2013;28:1953–60.
27. Imai A, Matsunami K, Takagi H, Ichigo S. Levonorgestrel-releasing intrauterine device used for dysmenorrhea: five-year literature review. Clin Exp Obstet Gynecol. 2014;41:495–8.

28. Croxatto HB. Clinical profile of Implanon: a single-rod etonogestrel contraceptive implant. Eur J Contracept Reprod Health Care. 2000;5(Suppl 2):21–8.
29. Walch K, et al. Implanon® versus medroxyprogesterone acetate: effects on pain scores in patients with symptomatic endometriosis—a pilot study. Contraception. 2009;79:29–34.
30. Dunselman GAJ, et al. ESHRE guideline: management of women with endometriosis. Hum Reprod. 2014;29:400–12.
31. Practice Bulletin No. 114: management of endometriosis. Obstet Gynecol. 2010;116:223–36.
32. Hughes E, et al. Ovulation suppression for endometriosis for women with subfertility. Cochrane Database Syst Rev. 2007;(3): CD000155. https://doi.org/10.1002/14651858.CD000155.pub2.
33. Bedaiwy M, Allaire C, Yong P, Alfaraj S. Medical management of endometriosis in patients with chronic pelvic pain. Semin Reprod Med. 2016;35:038–53.
34. Hickey M, Ballard K, Farquhar C. Endometriosis. BMJ. 2014;348:g1752.
35. Olive DL. Medical therapy of endometriosis. Semin Reprod Med. 2003;21:209–22.
36. Vercellini P, et al. Continuous use of an oral contraceptive for endometriosis-associated recurrent dysmenorrhea that does not respond to a cyclic pill regimen. Fertil Steril. 2003;80:560–3.
37. Harada T, Momoeda M, Taketani Y, Hoshiai H, Terakawa N. Low-dose oral contraceptive pill for dysmenorrhea associated with endometriosis: a placebo-controlled, double-blind, randomized trial. Fertil Steril. 2008;90:1583–8.
38. Muzii L, et al. Continuous versus cyclic oral contraceptives after laparoscopic excision of ovarian endometriomas: a systematic review and metaanalysis. Am J Obstet Gynecol. 2016;214:203–11.
39. Practice Committee of the American Society for Reproductive Medicine. Treatment of pelvic pain associated with endometriosis: a committee opinion. Fertil Steril. 2014;101:927–35.
40. Yisa SB, Okenwa AA, Husemeyer RP. Treatment of pelvic endometriosis with etonogestrel subdermal implant (Implanon®). J Fam Plann Reprod Health Care. 2005;31:67–9.
41. Maruo T, et al. Effects of the levonorgestrel-releasing intrauterine system on proliferation and apoptosis in the endometrium. Hum Reprod. 2001;16:2103–8.
42. Critchley HO, Wang H, Kelly RW, Gebbie AE, Glasier AF. Progestin receptor isoforms and prostaglandin dehydrogenase in the endometrium of women using a levonorgestrel-releasing intrauterine system. Hum Reprod. 1998;13:1210–7.
43. Vercellini P, et al. Comparison of a levonorgestrel-releasing intrauterine device versus expectant management after conservative surgery for symptomatic endometriosis: a pilot study. Fertil Steril. 2003;80:305–9.
44. Bayoglu Tekin Y, Dilbaz B, Altinbas SK, Dilbaz S. Postoperative medical treatment of chronic pelvic pain related to severe endometriosis: levonorgestrel-releasing intrauterine system versus gonadotropin-releasing hormone analogue. Fertil Steril. 2011;95:492–6.
45. Tanmahasamut P, et al. Postoperative levonorgestrel-releasing intrauterine system for pelvic endometriosis-related pain: a randomized controlled trial. Obstet Gynecol. 2012;119:519–26.
46. Charitidou C, et al. The administration of estrogens, combined with anti-androgens, has beneficial effects on the hormonal features and asymmetric dimethyl-arginine levels, in women with the polycystic ovary syndrome. Atherosclerosis. 2008;196:958–65.
47. Zimmerman Y, Eijkemans MJC, Coelingh Bennink HJT, Blankenstein MA, Fauser BCJM. The effect of combined oral contraception on testosterone levels in healthy women: a systematic review and meta-analysis. Hum Reprod Update. 2014;20:76–105.
48. Fauser BCJM, et al. Consensus on women's health aspects of polycystic ovary syndrome (PCOS): the Amsterdam ESHRE/ASRM-Sponsored 3rd PCOS Consensus Workshop Group. Fertil Steril. 2012;97:28–38.e25.
49. Elting MW, Korsen TJM, Bezemer PD, Schoemaker J. Prevalence of diabetes mellitus, hypertension and cardiac complaints in a follow-up study of a Dutch PCOS population. Hum Reprod. 2001;16:556–60.
50. Falsetti L, Gambera A, Tisi G. Efficacy of the combination ethinyl oestradiol and cyproterone acetate on endocrine, clinical and ultrasonographic profile in polycystic ovarian syndrome. Hum Reprod. 2001;16:36–42.

51. Venturoli S, et al. Ultrasound study of ovarian and uterine morphology in women with polycystic ovary syndrome before, during and after treatment with cyproterone acetate and ethinyloestradiol. Arch Gynecol. 1985;237:1–10.
52. Koltun W, Maloney JM, Marr J, Kunz M. Treatment of moderate acne vulgaris using a combined oral contraceptive containing ethinylestradiol 20μg plus drospirenone 3mg administered in a 24/4 regimen: a pooled analysis. Eur J Obstet Gynecol Reprod Biol. 2011;155:171–5.
53. Palombo-Kinne E, Schellschmidt I, Schumacher U, Gräser T. Efficacy of a combined oral contraceptive containing 0.030 mg ethinylestradiol/2 mg dienogest for the treatment of papulopustular acne in comparison with placebo and 0.035 mg ethinylestradiol/2 mg cyproterone acetate. Contraception. 2009;79:282–9.
54. Barnhart KT, Schreiber CA. Return to fertility following discontinuation of oral contraceptives. Fertil Steril. 2009;91:659–63.
55. Burke BM, Cunliffe WJ. Oral spironolactone therapy for female patients with acne, hirsutism or androgenic alopecia. Br J Dermatol. 1985;112:124–5.
56. Muhlemann MF, Carter GD, Cream JJ, Wise P. Oral spironolactone: an effective treatment for acne vulgaris in women. Br J Dermatol. 1986;115:227–32.
57. Loughlin J, et al. Risk of hyperkalemia in women taking ethinylestradiol/drospirenone and other oral contraceptives. Contraception. 2008;78:377–83.
58. Bird ST, et al. The association between drospirenone and hyperkalemia: a comparative-safety study. BMC Clin Pharmacol. 2011;11:23.
59. Mona Eng P, Seeger JD, Loughlin J, Oh K, Walker AM. Serum potassium monitoring for users of ethinyl estradiol/drospirenone taking medications predisposing to hyperkalemia: physician compliance and survey of knowledge and attitudes. Contraception. 2007;75:101–7.
60. Cagnacci A, et al. Menopause, estrogens, progestins, or their combination on body weight and anthropometric measures. Fertil Steril. 2007;88:1603–8.
61. Gierisch JM, et al. Oral contraceptive use and risk of breast, cervical, colorectal, and endometrial cancers: a systematic review. Cancer Epidemiol Biomarkers Prev. 2013;22:1931–43.
62. Iversen L, Sivasubramaniam S, Lee AJ, Fielding S, Hannaford PC. Lifetime cancer risk and combined oral contraceptives: the Royal College of General Practitioners' Oral Contraception Study. Am J Obstet Gynecol. 2017;216:580.e1–9.
63. Dossus L, et al. Reproductive risk factors and endometrial cancer: the European Prospective Investigation into Cancer and Nutrition. Int J Cancer. 2010;127(2):442–51. https://doi.org/10.1002/ijc.25050.
64. Havrilesky LJ, et al. Oral contraceptive pills as primary prevention for ovarian cancer: a systematic review and meta-analysis. Obstet Gynecol. 2013;122:139–47.
65. Jareid M, et al. Levonorgestrel-releasing intrauterine system use is associated with a decreased risk of ovarian and endometrial cancer, without increased risk of breast cancer. Results from the NOWAC Study. Gynecol Oncol. 2018;149:127–32.
66. Munro MG, Mainor N, Basu R, Brisinger M, Barreda L. Oral medroxyprogesterone acetate and combination oral contraceptives for acute uterine bleeding: a randomized controlled trial. Obstet Gynecol. 2006;108:924–9.
67. Haamid F, Sass AE, Dietrich JE. Heavy menstrual bleeding in adolescents. J Pediatr Adolesc Gynecol. 2017;30:335–40.
68. James AH, et al. Evaluation and management of acute menorrhagia in women with and without underlying bleeding disorders: consensus from an international expert panel. Eur J Obstet Gynecol Reprod Biol. 2011;158:124–34.
69. Desforges JF, Cowan BD, Morrison JC. Management of abnormal genital bleeding in girls and women. N Engl J Med. 1991;324:1710–5.
70. Santos M, Hendry D, Sangi-Haghpeykar H, Dietrich JE. Retrospective review of norethindrone use in adolescents. J Pediatr Adolesc Gynecol. 2014;27:41–4.
71. Portman DJ, et al. Efficacy and safety of an ascending-dose, extended-regimen levonorgestrel/ethinyl estradiol combined oral contraceptive. Contraception. 2014;89:299–306.

72. Traish AM, Vignozzi L, Simon JA, Goldstein I, Kim NN. Role of androgens in female genitourinary tissue structure and function: implications in the genitourinary syndrome of menopause. Sex Med Rev. 2018;6:558–71.
73. Davis SR, Braunstein GD. Efficacy and safety of testosterone in the management of hypoactive sexual desire disorder in postmenopausal women. J Sex Med. 2012;9:1134–48.
74. Coelingh Bennink HJT, et al. Maintaining physiological testosterone levels by adding dehydroepiandrosterone to combined oral contraceptives: I. Endocrine effects. Contraception. 2017;96:322–9.
75. van Lunsen RHW, et al. Maintaining physiologic testosterone levels during combined oral contraceptives by adding dehydroepiandrosterone: II. Effects on sexual function. A phase II randomized, double-blind, placebo-controlled study. Contraception. 2018;98:56–62.
76. Mawet M, et al. Unique effects on hepatic function, lipid metabolism, bone and growth endocrine parameters of estetrol in combined oral contraceptives. Eur J Contracept Reprod Health Care. 2015;20:463–75.
77. Kluft C, et al. Reduced hemostatic effects with drospirenone-based oral contraceptives containing estetrol vs. ethinyl estradiol. Contraception. 2017;95:140–7.
78. Duijkers IJM, et al. Inhibition of ovulation by administration of estetrol in combination with drospirenone or levonorgestrel: results of a phase II dose-finding pilot study. Eur J Contracept Reprod Health Care. 2015;20:476–89.

Heavy Menstrual Bleeding in Adolescents

Laura Gaspari, Francoise Paris, Nicolas Kalfa, and Charles Sultan

Heavy or prolonged or frequent menstrual bleeding at menarche is a common concern in adolescent and can be an important sentinel for an underlying bleeding disorder [1–3].

L. Gaspari
CHU Montpellier, Université de Montpellier, Unité d'Endocrinologie-Gynécologie Pédiatrique, Service de Pédiatrie, Montpellier, France

CHU Montpellier, Université de Montpellier, Centre de Référence Maladies Rares du Développement Génital, Constitutif Sud, Hôpital Lapeyronie, Montpellier, France

F. Paris
CHU Montpellier, Université de Montpellier, Unité d'Endocrinologie-Gynécologie Pédiatrique, Service de Pédiatrie, Montpellier, France

CHU Montpellier, Université de Montpellier, Centre de Référence Maladies Rares du Développement Génital, Constitutif Sud, Hôpital Lapeyronie, Montpellier, France

Université de Montpellier, INSERM 1203, DEFE, Montpellier, France
e-mail: f-paris@chu-montpellier.fr

N. Kalfa
CHU Montpellier, Université de Montpellier, Centre de Référence Maladies Rares du Développement Génital, Constitutif Sud, Hôpital Lapeyronie, Montpellier, France

Université de Montpellier, INSERM 1203, DEFE, Montpellier, France

CHU Montpellier, Université de Montpellier, Département de Chirurgie Pédiatrique, Hôpital Lapeyronie, Montpellier, France
e-mail: n-kalfa@chu-montpellier.fr

C. Sultan (✉)
CHU Montpellier, Université de Montpellier, Unité d'Endocrinologie-Gynécologie Pédiatrique, Service de Pédiatrie, Montpellier, France

© The Author(s), under exclusive license to Springer Nature Switzerland AG 2024
A. R. Genazzani et al. (eds.), *Menstrual Bleeding and Pain Disorders from Adolescence to Menopause*, ISGE Series,
https://doi.org/10.1007/978-3-031-55300-4_3

In this overview, we will discuss the recent changes made by experts to standardize nomenclature and definition of heavy menstrual bleeding (HMB), we will report helpful tools to diagnose HMB, and we will present the causes and will discuss the medical management of this menstrual disorder in adolescents.

1   Definition

Heavy menstrual bleeding (HMB) refers to uterine bleeding that is abnormal in volume, frequency, duration and regularity and that occurs mostly in the menarcheal period. HMB is a common gynaecological complaint in adolescents and can be a source of distress and morbidity [4]. HMB is a confusing and freighting event for the adolescents and their family [5, 6]. It may lead to lower perceived female health and poor quality of life and may affect participation in school, sports and other activities. Its prevalence ranges between 27% in American adolescents and 37% in Swedish adolescents [7, 8].

According to the International Federation of Gynaecology and Obstetrics (FIGO), HMB can be defined as "excessive menstrual blood loss that interferes with a woman's normal physical, emotional, social and material quality of life, and that can occur alone or in combination with other symptoms" [9, 10]. Changes have been made to standardize nomenclature and classification of abnormal uterine bleeding in adolescents [11]. HMB must replace previously used terms, such as menorrhagia, metrorrhagia, polymenorrhagia, dysfunctional uterine bleeding, abnormal uterine bleeding and heavy and prolonged menstrual bleeding [12, 13].

Girls with prolonged HMB should be referred to paediatricians and/or gynaecologists specialized in adolescent health and/or haematologists when an underlying bleeding disorder is suspected [14, 15].

2   The Menstrual Cycle at Puberty

The normal menstrual cycle is divided into proliferative, ovulatory and secretary phase. Menstruation occurs when the endometrium collapses and sheds following the rapid decline in progesterone concentration. Then, menstrual flow stops as a result of the combined effects of vasoconstriction and vascular stasis.

In abnormal menstrual cycles, progesterone deficiency and suboptimal oestrogen levels are associated with intermittent heavy bleeding. According to the American College of Obstetricians and Gynecologists (ACOG) and the Association of Applied Biologists (AAB), the menstrual cycle should be considered as a vital sign [16] because abnormal cycles can reflect hypothalamic-pituitary-ovarian axis dysfunction, general diseases or iatrogenic problems [8, 17]. The normal menstrual cycle usually lasts ~28 days (±5 days). The mean menstrual flow duration is 4 days

(±2 days), and the normal blood loss is approximately 30 mL per cycle, with an upper limit of 60–70 mL.

The monthly menstrual flow largely depends on the proper functioning of the hypothalamic-pituitary-ovarian axis and of the haemostatic system. During the first year after menarche, abnormal and/or irregular bleeding should be considered as part of the normal pubertal immaturity of the hypothalamic-pituitary-ovarian axis. If HMB persists when menstrual cycles become regular, other HMB causes should be ruled out.

3   Diagnosis

In most cases, HMB occurs during the first years after menarche. Therefore, it is mandatory to determine the age at menarche. The initial goal in an adolescent with HMB is to evaluate the haemodynamic stability and to identify whether bleeding is associated with ovulatory dysfunction or with an underlying coagulation disorder. The diagnosis is based on the patient's menstrual history, bleeding history, family history of bleeding disorders, physical examination and laboratory investigations.

3.1   Menstrual History

An accurate and complete menstrual history is critical. Precise questions should focus on the cycle length, period length and quality (e.g. flooding). For this, it is important to determine the number of sanitary pads or tampons used per day and the presence of blood clots. The use of a structured chart can be sometimes helpful (e.g. pictorial blood assessment chart) [18].

HMB is defined by the following:

– Menstrual cycle >45 days or <21 days
– Menstrual bleeding >7 days
– Blood loss >80 mL/day

3.2   Bleeding History

If HMB occurs at menarche onset, an underlying coagulation disorder should be suspected. Special attention should be paid to symptoms, such as epistaxis lasting more than 10 min and prolonged bleeding after minor wounds/tooth extraction (Table 1) [19, 20]. Moreover, it should be determined whether HMB negatively affects the perceived general health, quality of life and participation in school, sports and social activities [21].

Table 1 Conditions that should lead to suspect an underlying bleeding disorder in adolescents with HMB

1. Menses lasting >7 days
2. Menstrual flow that requires >5 sanitary pads or tampons per day
3. Passage of large blood clots
4. Failure to respond to conventional therapy
5. Family history of bleeding symptoms
6. Heavy menstrual bleeding since menarche
7. One of the following signs:
• Surgery-related haemorrhage
• Bleeding associated with dental procedures or tooth extraction
8. Two or more of the following symptoms:
• Bruising with minimal or no trauma, once or twice per month
• Epistaxis lasting >10 min, once or twice per month
• Frequent gum bleeding
• Prolonged bleeding from trivial wounds lasting >15 min

3.3 Family History

A detailed familial history of bleeding symptoms should be obtained. It is important to identify a family history of bleeding disorders, unexpected haemorrhages or frequent blood transfusions.

3.4 Physical Examination

HMB is a common cause of iron deficiency and anaemia that are associated with poor concentration, restless legs and fatigue [22–24]. In some cases, HMB requires admission to an intensive care unit. Physical examination should begin with vital signs, such as tachycardia, orthostatic hypotension and conjunctival pallor. The skin should be inspected for petechiae and purpura, which are considered physical signs of a bleeding disorder, and pale colouring. Weight and body mass index should be recorded. Signs of androgen excess, such as acne and hirsutism, should also be investigated.

3.5 Laboratory Investigations

When a bleeding disorder is suspected, the adolescent health specialist should work in collaboration with a haematologist to interpret the laboratory data and propose new investigations, if needed [5, 25, 26]. The routine laboratory work-up must include (Table 2):

– Complete blood count to screen for anaemia and thrombocytopaenia
– Haemoglobin and ferritin levels

Table 2 Haematologic work-up for haemostasis disorders, according to Borzutzky et al. [26]

1. Platelet evaluation
• Complete blood cell count
• Platelet function assay (PFA-100)
• Platelet aggregation
2. Von Willebrand disease evaluation
• Von Willebrand factor antigen (vWF:Ag)
• Factor VIII activity
• Von Willebrand factor multimers
3. Collagen evaluation
• Platelet aggregation
• Hypermobility score
4. Coagulation factors
• Prothrombin time
• Activated partial thromboplastin time
• Factor XIII assay
5. Fibrinogen evaluation
• Prothrombin time
• Activated partial thromboplastin time
• Fibrinogen assay

- Prothrombin time, activated partial thromboplastin time and bleeding time to detect blood dyscrasia and coagulation disorders
- Von Willebrand factor antigen and factor VIII
- Testing for sexually transmitted infections

3.6 Pelvic Ultrasound

In a retrospective study on 230 adolescents with HMB, Pechiolli et al. analysed the pelvic ultrasound imaging data and HMB management [27]. They found that pelvic ultrasound is not required for the initial evaluation of HMB because it did not influence treatment decision-making.

4 HMB Causes

According to the FIGO recommendations adapted from Munro et al., HMB can be related to structural and non-structural causes [10]. Structural causes of HMB include polyps, adenomyosis, leiomyoma, malignancy and hyperplasia; non-structural causes of HMB are related to coagulopathy, ovulatory dysfunction, endometrial, iatrogenic and not yet classified factors [10]. Ovulatory dysfunction is the leading cause of HMB (~90% of all HMB cases) [8]. Other HMB causes are coagulation disorders, endocrine diseases, benign lesions of the genital tract and side effects of several drugs (Table 3).

Table 3 Main causes of HMB, according to Kabra et al. [5, 8]

1. Ovulatory dysfunction
2. Coagulopathies
• Thrombocytopenia
• Von Willebrand diseases
– Type 1: quantitative deficiency of vWF
– Type 2: qualitative defect in vWF activity
– Type 3: absent vWF
• Glanzmann thromboasthenia: anomaly of the platelet membrane glycoproteins IIb or IIIa
• Bernard-Soulier syndrome: inherited deficiency in platelet membrane Ib-IX glycoprotein complex
3. Endocrine diseases
• Hyperandrogenism: polycystic ovarian syndrome
• Thyroid dysfunction
• Adrenal disease (Cushing syndrome)
• Hyperprolactaemia
• Primary ovarian insufficiency
4. Utero-vaginal diseases
• Polyps
• Adenomyosis
• Endometritis
5. Infections
• Pelvic inflammatory disease
• Cervicitis, vaginitis
6. Medications
• Hormonal therapy
• Anabolic steroids
• Chemo-/radiotherapy
• Antipsychotic, antidepressants
• Anticonvulsivants
7. Trauma
8. Stress

4.1 Ovulatory Dysfunction

Peri-pubertal immaturity of the hypothalamic-pituitary-ovarian axis is characterized by the absence of the ovulatory luteinizing hormone surge. Follicular atresia and lack of progesterone production lead to an unopposed estrogenic proliferation of the endometrium, amplified through obesity, early menarche and estrogenic endocrine disruptor contamination, followed by its irregular shedding that causes the abnormal bleeding [28]. There is general consensus that in the first gynaecological years, the majority of menstrual cycles are anovulatory. Indeed, in a recent meta-analysis, Carlson et al. reported that only 48% of girls present ovulatory cycles at gynaecological age of 3 years and 60% of them present ovulatory cycles at gynaecological age of 5 years [29]. When abnormal cycles persist after more than 3 years post-menarche, more investigations are needed [7, 8].

4.2 Coagulation Disorders

Inherited or acquired bleeding disorders, such as von Willebrand disease, and quantitative and qualitative platelet abnormalities are common findings in adolescents with HMB and require specialized laboratory investigations (Table 2) [30, 31].

4.3 Endocrine Diseases

Hyperandrogenism and polycystic syndrome, hypercortisolism, thyroid dysfunctions, obesity and anorexia nervosa, excess exercise and stress may be associated with HMB [32].

4.4 Iatrogenic Causes

It has been reported that progesterone-only contraceptive methods cause HMB. In some adolescents, also combined oral contraceptives are associated with HMB in the first months of use. Anabolic steroids, corticosteroids, anticoagulants, anticonvulsants and anti-inflammatory drugs also can cause HMB.

4.5 Structural Causes

Endometrium/uterus abnormalities (adenomyosis, endometriosis and cervical polyps) are uncommon causes of HMB and are rather associated with pain during regular cycles.

5 HMB Management

A multidisciplinary approach is needed in which gynaecologists, paediatricians and haematologists work together to provide a personalized management for each adolescent (Table 4) [33]. In some patients, HMB is not a significant health concern [34]. However, in the case of acute haemorrhage and anaemia, adolescents may require emergency hospital admission [35]. HMB unrelated to uterine structure

Table 4 HMB management, according to Moon et al. [7, 33]

1. Blood transfusion if the patient has symptomatic severe anaemia and Hb < 9 g/dL
2. Iron supplementation in the presence of iron deficiency or iron deficiency anaemia (60–120 mg/day)
3. Conjugated equine oestrogen (Premarin): 25 mg intravenous every 4–6 h, 4 times
4. Combined oral contraceptives
• 50 μg ethinyl oestradiol combined contraceptive pill every 6–8 h for 1 week, then reduced every week down to daily dosing
• 30–35 μg ethinyl oestradiol combined monophasic contraceptive pill, every 6–8 h for 1 week, then reduced to daily dosing
5. Progestins:
• Medroxyprogesterone acetate (Provera), per os, 10–20 mg, every 6–8 h, for 1 week, then reduced to daily dosing
• Norethindrone: 5–15 mg/day
6. Levonorgestrel intrauterine device (52 mg)
7. Desmopressin: synthetic vasopressin analogue that stimulates the release of von Willebrand factor
8. Tranexamic acid
• 10 mg/kg intravenous every 6–8 h, for 2–5 days
• 180 mg per os every 8 h, for 5 days
9. Non-steroidal anti-inflammatory drugs
• Ibuprofen, 600–800 mg, every 6–8 h

abnormalities are amenable to medical management, whereas HMB caused by uterine abnormalities require surgical management.

The goals of HMB management are:

- To stop bleeding
- To restore adequate estrogenic levels and endometrium synchrony
- To restore iron levels [36, 37]
- To prevent complications

Management should be tailored in function of the clinical presentation and laboratory results. HMB is usually classified into three groups, according to the patient's haemoglobin (Hb) levels:

- Mild HMB: Hb >11 g/dL
- Moderate HMB: Hb = 9–11 g/dL
- Severe HMB: Hb < 9 g/dL

Routinely, Hb level of 9 g/dL is considered the threshold for treatment decision-making:

- If Hb < 9 g/dL, the adolescent requires emergency and intensive treatment:

  - Conjugated oestrogens (e.g. Premarin, per os, intramuscular or intravenous)
  - Progestins: progesterone depot injection or per os
  - Oral contraceptives: Desogestrel is the most prescribed

- Non-steroidal anti-inflammatory drugs: ibuprofen
- Antifibrinolytic agents: Amicar
- Iron supplementation: ferrous sulphate

- If Hb > 9 g/dL:

  - Oral contraceptive pill, cyclical progestogens should be prescribed.
  - Iron supplementation is usually offered.

6 Conclusions

HMB should be considered as a part of normal pubertal development rather than a disease [38]. The majority of adolescents with HMB will thus spontaneously convert to normal menstrual cycle within 3–4 years after menarche. Overall, adolescents with HMB have an excellent prognosis. For those with underlying bleeding disorders, the prognosis depends on the haematological cause.

In conclusion, although HMB should be considered as a sign of the physiological process of maturation of the hypothalamic-pituitary-ovarian axis, it may affect the adolescent's quality of life and social life. Moreover, a correct evaluation of menstrual disturbances is a good opportunity to detect a hypothalamic-pituitary-ovarian axis dysfunction or an underlying coagulation defect.

References

1. Bennett AR, Gray SH. What to do when she's bleeding through: the recognition, evaluation, and management of abnormal uterine bleeding in adolescents. Curr Opin Pediatr. 2014;26(4):413–9. https://doi.org/10.1097/MOP.0000000000000121.
2. Emans SJH, Laufer MR, DiVasta AD. Goldstein's pediatric & adolescent gynecology. 7th ed. Wolters Kluwer; 2020.
3. Haamid F, Sass AE, Dietrich JE. Heavy menstrual bleeding in adolescents. J Pediatr Adolesc Gynecol. 2017;30(3):335–40. https://doi.org/10.1016/j.jpag.2017.01.002.
4. Schoep ME, Nieboer TE, van der Zanden M, Braat DDM, Nap AW. The impact of menstrual symptoms on everyday life: a survey among 42,879 women. Am J Obstet Gynecol. 2019;220(6):569.e1–7. https://doi.org/10.1016/j.ajog.2019.02.048.
5. Screening and management of bleeding disorders in adolescents with heavy menstrual bleeding: ACOG COMMITTEE OPINION, Number 785. Obstet Gynecol. 2019;134(3):e71–83. https://doi.org/10.1097/AOG.0000000000003411.
6. Committee on Practice B-G. Practice bulletin no. 128: diagnosis of abnormal uterine bleeding in reproductive-aged women. Obstet Gynecol. 2012;120(1):197–206. https://doi.org/10.1097/AOG.0b013e318262e320.
7. Moon LM, Perez-Milicua G, Dietrich JE. Evaluation and management of heavy menstrual bleeding in adolescents. Curr Opin Obstet Gynecol. 2017;29(5):328–36. https://doi.org/10.1097/GCO.0000000000000394.
8. Kabra R, Fisher M. Abnormal uterine bleeding in adolescents. Curr Probl Pediatr Adolesc Health Care. 2022;52(5):101185. https://doi.org/10.1016/j.cppeds.2022.101185.

9. Munro MG, Critchley H, Fraser IS. Research and clinical management for women with abnormal uterine bleeding in the reproductive years: more than PALM-COEIN. BJOG. 2017;124(2):185–9. https://doi.org/10.1111/1471-0528.14431.

10. Munro MG, Critchley HOD, Fraser IS, Committee FMD. The two FIGO systems for normal and abnormal uterine bleeding symptoms and classification of causes of abnormal uterine bleeding in the reproductive years: 2018 revisions. Int J Gynaecol Obstet. 2018;143(3):393–408. https://doi.org/10.1002/ijgo.12666.

11. Chodankar RR, Munro MG, Critchley HOD. Historical perspectives and evolution of menstrual terminology. Front Reprod Health. 2022;4:820029. https://doi.org/10.3389/frph.2022.820029.

12. Fraser IS, Critchley HO, Broder M, Munro MG. The FIGO recommendations on terminologies and definitions for normal and abnormal uterine bleeding. Semin Reprod Med. 2011;29(5):383–90. https://doi.org/10.1055/s-0031-1287662.

13. Excellence NIfHaC: Heavy menstrual bleeding: assessment and management (NICE guideline NG88). Accessed 14 Mar 2018.

14. O'Brien SH. Evaluation and management of heavy menstrual bleeding in adolescents: the role of the hematologist. Blood. 2018;132(20):2134–42. https://doi.org/10.1182/blood-2018-05-848739.

15. Dickerson KE, Menon NM, Zia A. Abnormal uterine bleeding in young women with blood disorders. Pediatr Clin N Am. 2018;65(3):543–60. https://doi.org/10.1016/j.pcl.2018.02.008.

16. ACOG Committee Opinion No. 651: menstruation in girls and adolescents: using the menstrual cycle as a vital sign. Obstet Gynecol. 2015;126(6):e143–6. https://doi.org/10.1097/AOG.0000000000001215.

17. Hennegan J, Winkler IT, Bobel C, Keiser D, Hampton J, Larsson G, et al. Menstrual health: a definition for policy, practice, and research. Sex Reprod Health Matters. 2021;29(1):1911618. https://doi.org/10.1080/26410397.2021.1911618.

18. Higham JM, O'Brien PM, Shaw RW. Assessment of menstrual blood loss using a pictorial chart. Br J Obstet Gynaecol. 1990;97(8):734–9. https://doi.org/10.1111/j.1471-0528.1990.tb16249.x.

19. Quint EH, Smith YR. Abnormal uterine bleeding in adolescents. J Midwifery Womens Health. 2003;48(3):186–91. https://doi.org/10.1016/s1526-9523(03)00061-8.

20. Davila J, Alderman EM. Heavy menstrual bleeding in adolescent girls. Pediatr Ann. 2020;49(4):e163–e9. https://doi.org/10.3928/19382359-20200321-01.

21. Nur Azurah AG, Sanci L, Moore E, Grover S. The quality of life of adolescents with menstrual problems. J Pediatr Adolesc Gynecol. 2013;26(2):102–8. https://doi.org/10.1016/j.jpag.2012.11.004.

22. Camaschella C. Iron deficiency: new insights into diagnosis and treatment. Hematology Am Soc Hematol Educ Program. 2015;2015:8–13. https://doi.org/10.1182/asheducation-2015.1.8.

23. Johnson S, Lang A, Sturm M, O'Brien SH. Iron deficiency without anemia: a common yet under-recognized diagnosis in young women with heavy menstrual bleeding. J Pediatr Adolesc Gynecol. 2016;29(6):628–31. https://doi.org/10.1016/j.jpag.2016.05.009.

24. Mansour D, Hofmann A, Gemzell-Danielsson K. A review of clinical guidelines on the management of iron deficiency and iron-deficiency anemia in women with heavy menstrual bleeding. Adv Ther. 2021;38(1):201–25. https://doi.org/10.1007/s12325-020-01564-y.

25. Zia A, Rajpurkar M. Challenges of diagnosing and managing the adolescent with heavy menstrual bleeding. Thromb Res. 2016;143:91–100. https://doi.org/10.1016/j.thromres.2016.05.001.

26. Borzutzky C, Jaffray J. Diagnosis and management of heavy menstrual bleeding and bleeding disorders in adolescents. JAMA Pediatr. 2020;174(2):186–94. https://doi.org/10.1001/jamapediatrics.2019.5040.

27. Pecchioli Y, Oyewumi L, Allen LM, Kives S. The utility of routine ultrasound in the diagnosis and management of adolescents with abnormal uterine bleeding. J Pediatr Adolesc Gynecol. 2017;30(2):239–42. https://doi.org/10.1016/j.jpag.2016.09.012.

28. Jain V, Chodankar RR, Maybin JA, Critchley HOD. Uterine bleeding: how understanding endometrial physiology underpins menstrual health. Nat Rev Endocrinol. 2022;18(5):290–308. https://doi.org/10.1038/s41574-021-00629-4.
29. Carlson LJ, Shaw ND. Development of ovulatory menstrual cycles in adolescent girls. J Pediatr Adolesc Gynecol. 2019;32(3):249–53. https://doi.org/10.1016/j.jpag.2019.02.119.
30. Rajpurkar M, O'Brien SH, Haamid FW, Cooper DL, Gunawardena S, Chitlur M. Heavy menstrual bleeding as a common presenting symptom of rare platelet disorders: illustrative case examples. J Pediatr Adolesc Gynecol. 2016;29(6):537–41. https://doi.org/10.1016/j.jpag.2016.02.002.
31. Zia A, Stanek J, Christian-Rancy M, Ahuja SP, Savelli S, O'Brien SH. Utility of a screening tool for haemostatic defects in a multicentre cohort of adolescents with heavy menstrual bleeding. Haemophilia. 2018;24(6):957–63. https://doi.org/10.1111/hae.13609.
32. Matthews ML. Abnormal uterine bleeding in reproductive-aged women. Obstet Gynecol Clin N Am. 2015;42(1):103–15. https://doi.org/10.1016/j.ogc.2014.09.006.
33. Powers JM, Stanek JR, Srivaths L, Haamid FW, O'Brien SH. Hematologic considerations and management of adolescent girls with heavy menstrual bleeding and anemia in US children's hospitals. J Pediatr Adolesc Gynecol. 2018;31(5):446–50. https://doi.org/10.1016/j.jpag.2018.06.008.
34. Alaqzam TS, Stanley AC, Simpson PM, Flood VH, Menon S. Treatment modalities in adolescents who present with heavy menstrual bleeding. J Pediatr Adolesc Gynecol. 2018;31(5):451–8. https://doi.org/10.1016/j.jpag.2018.02.130.
35. Bradley LD, Gueye NA. The medical management of abnormal uterine bleeding in reproductive-aged women. Am J Obstet Gynecol. 2016;214(1):31–44. https://doi.org/10.1016/j.ajog.2015.07.044.
36. Percy L, Mansour D, Fraser I. Iron deficiency and iron deficiency anaemia in women. Best Pract Res Clin Obstet Gynaecol. 2017;40:55–67. https://doi.org/10.1016/j.bpobgyn.2016.09.007.
37. Munro MG, FIGO Committee on Menstrual Disorders. Abnormal uterine bleeding: a well-travelled path to iron deficiency and anemia. Int J Gynaecol Obstet. 2020;150(3):275–7. https://doi.org/10.1002/ijgo.13180.
38. Luiro K, Holopainen E. Heavy menstrual bleeding in adolescent: normal or a sign of an underlying disease? Semin Reprod Med. 2022;40(1-02):23–31. https://doi.org/10.1055/s-0041-1739309.

The Correlation Between Abnormal Uterine Bleeding in Early Menarche and PCOS Later in Adolescence

Efthymios Deligeoroglou and Vasileios Karountzos

1 Introduction

Abnormal uterine bleeding (AUB) includes a variety of symptoms in adolescence. Among these are heavy menstrual bleeding, intermenstrual bleeding, and the simultaneous existence of heavy and prolonged menstrual bleeding [1]. Up to 14% of women during their reproductive years will report AUB at least one time during their lifetime, with subsequent physical, emotional, sexual, social, and financial problems [2, 3]. The International Federation of Gynecology and Obstetrics (FIGO) Menstrual Disorders Working Group proposed a new classification system for the diagnosis of AUB in non-gravid women of reproductive age in 2011 which since been adopted worldwide [1]. This classification has been also accepted by the American College of Obstetricians and Gynecologists (ACOG). Specifically, FIGO suggested the term PALM-COEIN, which stands for the following causes of AUB: polyp, adenomyosis, leiomyoma, malignancy and hyperplasia, coagulopathy, ovulatory dysfunction, endometrial, iatrogenic, and not otherwise classified [1].

In otherwise healthy adolescents, the most common cause of AUB (more than 95% of cases) is anovulation [4]. The immaturity of the hypothalamic-pituitary-ovarian (HPO) axis accounts for the vast majority of these cases, but there are also other endocrine disorders associated with anovulation. The most common of these

E. Deligeoroglou (✉)
Pediatric and Adolescent Gynecology, Medical School, National and Kapodistrian University of Athens, Athens, Greece

Division of Pediatric-Adolescent Gynecology, "MITERA" Children's Hospital, Athens, Greece

V. Karountzos
Division of Pediatric-Adolescent Gynecology, "MITERA" Children's Hospital, Athens, Greece

A. R. Genazzani et al. (eds.), *Menstrual Bleeding and Pain Disorders from Adolescence to Menopause*, ISGE Series,
https://doi.org/10.1007/978-3-031-55300-4_4

endocrinopathies is polycystic ovarian syndrome (PCOS) [4]. Practitioners should always remember that before making the diagnosis of AUB in adolescence, due to anovulation, several other underlying pathologies such as bleeding disorders (e.g., von Willebrand Disease), pathologies of the reproductive tract (e.g., polyps), trauma, pregnancy, medication, as well as other endocrine disorders (e.g., hypothyroidism) must also be taken under consideration [4].

Since PCOS is the most common endocrine disorder during adolescence, there is an obvious correlation between this endocrinologic disorder and the symptom of AUB. The criteria, which are used for its diagnosis, will affect its prevalence, which is between 10% and 20% [5]. Even though many years have passed from when syndrome was first reported, the pathophysiology, as well as the age of onset of PCOS, is not yet fully understood, while the establishment of worldwide accepted diagnostic criteria remains a challenge. Hyperandrogenism, chronic anovulation, and infertility are the main features of this heterogeneous condition. The National Institute of Health (NIH) recommends that the diagnostic criteria for PCOS should comprise the concomitant presence of anovulation and evidence of hyperandrogenemia—biochemical, clinical (hirsutism/acne), or both—irrespective of ovarian morphology, while the Androgen Excess Society proposed that hyperandrogenism should be a presupposition for the diagnosis of the syndrome, together with ovarian dysfunction, expressed as chronic anovulation or polycystic ovarian morphology on ultrasound [5, 6]. The European Society of Human Reproduction and Embryology/American Society for Reproductive Medicine proposed the Rotterdam criteria (ESHRE/ASRM) [7, 8], in which the diagnosis is established when two out of three of the following criteria are met, in the absence of other known etiologies: anovulation or oligo-ovulation, clinical and/or biochemical hyperandrogenism, and polycystic ovaries by ultrasound (US). These three diagnostic approaches are widely used to date.

2 Menarche and Normal Menstrual Cycle

Median age at menarche has remained relatively stable in the last 10 years worldwide, between 12 and 13 years, with variations between well-nourished populations in developed countries [9]. Menarche typically occurs within 2–3 years after thelarche, at Tanner stage IV breast development, and is rare before Tanner stage III development. By age 15 years, 98% of females will have had menarche [10]. In the first gynecological year of the adolescent girl, the cycle interval is between 21 and 45 days (mean, 32.2 days), and the flow length is usually about 7 days. As the years pass from menarche, the menstrual cycle usually normalizes with more regular cycles, and by the third year after menarche, 60–80% of menstrual cycles are between 21 and 34 days [11].

The HPO axis plays the most crucial role in normal menstrual cycle. It is well known, in the follicular phase of the menstrual cycle, follicle-stimulating hormone (FSH) acts on ovarian follicles, and estrogen is produced by granulosa cells. By day

5–7 a dominant follicle appears, leading to another rise in the estrogen level with subsequent growth of the endometrium. This estrogenic rise acts as a negative feedback to FSH, at the same time that stimulates a surge in luteinizing hormone (LH), which leads to ovulation. In the second phase of the cycle, the remaining corpus luteum produces progesterone, making the endometrium secretory, and in the absence of fertilization, progesterone and estrogen levels fall rapidly, leading to shedding of the endometrial lining [11].

3   Physiological Adolescent Anovulation

As previously discussed before, the menstrual cycle is established in most adolescents 3 years after menarche. Thus more than 50% of menstrual cycles are anovulatory before this time. Anovulation is expressed either with oligomenorrhea or AUB. Girls who are less than 12 years of age at menarche have 50% ovulatory cycles by 1 year after menarche, whereas girls with onset of menarche at 12–13 years of age or greater than 13 years need 3 or sometimes 4–5 years, respectively, to establish 50% ovulatory cycles [12]. Although ovulatory dysfunction is somewhat physiologic in the first few years after menarche, it can be associated with endocrinopathies due to HPO axis disturbances, such as PCOS [1]. Although the diagnosis of PCOS should not be established in the first years after menarche, the presence of AUB with a PCOS-like increase in LH levels and pulse frequency, as well as with a significantly higher plasma testosterone, may be the first signs postmenarchal of a subsequent PCOS diagnosis [13, 14]. Therefore, anovulation, which persists more than 2 years, predicts many future PCOS cases, while insulin resistance, which can be physiologically seen in puberty, is like that of PCOS in its degree and in its tissue selectivity [15, 16]. Finally, it is also well known that the ovary of postmenarchal anovulatory adolescent has histologically polycystic morphology.

4   Pathophysiology of AUB

As mentioned above, more of 95% of AUB cases are due to anovulation based on the absence of LH surge in menstrual cycle. The cause of this absence is that the positive feedback of estradiol to LH is not working as it should. If increasing levels of estrogen do not cause a decrease in follicle-stimulating hormone (FSH) secretion with subsequent suppression of estrogen secretion, multiple follicular recruitment is stimulated, and a dominant follicle does not form. As a result, corpus luteum is not observed, and follicular atresia is unavoidable, leading to cystic formation, producing only estrogens and not progesterone [4]. The target organ of this process is the uterus, in which endometrial proliferation is observed, due to unopposed estrogen. Even though the endometrium is thick, it starts shedding irregularly resulting in blood loss, due to absence of progesterone stabilization [17, 18]. Such heavy bleeding may be worsened by an increase in prostacyclin synthesis in endometrial capillary epithelial cells under the influence of estrogens in the absence of progesterone.

On the other hand, there are adolescents who experience AUB even when ovulating. In these cases, the HPO axis works normally, but there is an imbalance between the vasoconstrictive effect of PGF2a and vasodilation of PGE2 and PGI2 (prostacyclin), while the circulating steroid levels act synergistically in endometrial PG production. Total PG and PGE2 levels have been observed to be elevated in ovulatory AUB [19].

5 Causes of AUB

There are several causes that should be excluded before making the diagnosis of anovulatory AUB, due to immaturity of the HPO axis. Use of PALM-COEIN should be the basis of the differential diagnosis, but also other conditions should be taken under consideration as shown in Fig. 1. Some of them may be overlapping the PALM-COEIN acronym, and some of them require immediate exclusion because failure to do so may result in significant morbidity and mortality [15]. Pregnancy-related complications can present with any pattern of abnormal bleeding, and among them ectopic pregnancy is one of the more serious conditions to be considered. Endocrine disorders should always be at the top of the differential diagnosis of AUB

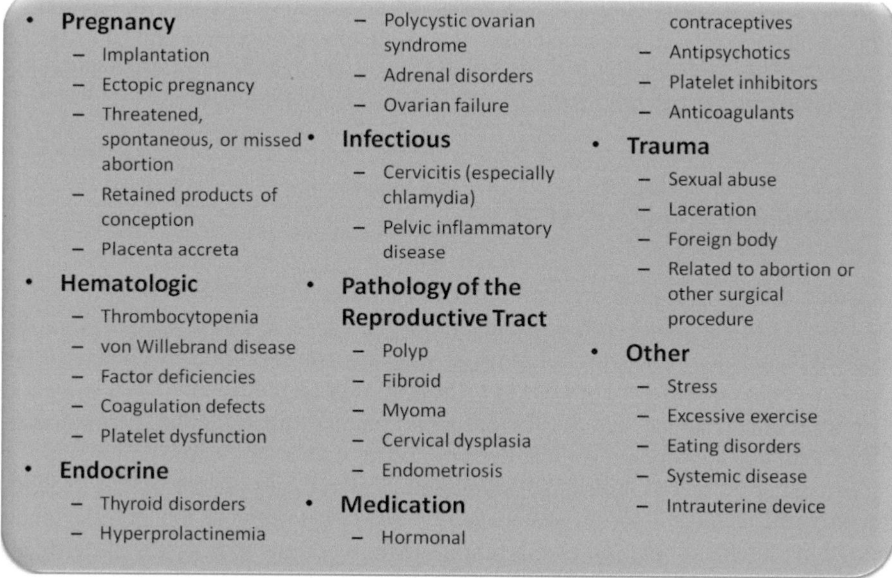

Fig. 1 Differential diagnosis of AUB in adolescents. (Adapted by [4])

with PCOS and thyroid disorders being very common, while others such as hyperprolactinemia should always be evaluated. If clinically indicated, adrenal gland abnormalities, such as Addison's disease, late-onset congenital adrenal hyperplasia, or Cushing's disease, may also need to be excluded [4, 20]. Adolescents with pelvic inflammatory disease (PID) and endometritis caused by *Neisseria gonorrhoeae* or *Chlamydia trachomatis*, frequently present with heavy or irregular bleeding. PID may present with vaginal bleeding in addition to lower abdominal pain, especially in sexually active adolescents [15]. Moreover, the possibility of a coagulopathy should be kept in mind, particularly in the adolescent whose menstrual history is short and not yet well defined. More than a third of adolescents may have a coagulation defect [16, 17]. Bleeding disorders are usually associated with cyclic heavy or prolonged bleeding (menorrhagia). We consider the possibility of a bleeding disorder (coagulation factor deficiency or inherited or acquired platelet disorder) in adolescents who present with first menses with extremely heavy flow, bleeding requiring blood transfusion or hospitalization, and patients with refractory heavy menstrual bleeding and concomitant anemia. In such patients, consultation with a hematologist is warranted. In retrospective studies in adolescents hospitalized for heavy menstrual bleeding, the prevalence of bleeding disorders ranges from 5% to 28%. The same pattern may be observed in women receiving treatment with anticoagulants [18, 19]. In addition, severe thrombocytopenia can be assessed quickly with a complete blood cell count. The possibility of an underlying abnormality is high, if an adolescent has to be hospitalized and her hemoglobin is less than 10 g/dL [17]. Although adult women commonly present with an underlying pathology, such as fibroids, dysplasia, or cancer, adolescents rarely present with such conditions. However, these conditions are sometimes seen in young women and should be considered during the differential diagnosis of abnormal bleeding [15]. Furthermore, a variety of different medications can predispose to abnormal bleeding, including glucocorticoids, tamoxifen, and anticoagulants. Intermenstrual bleeding is a common side effect of oral contraceptives, depot medroxyprogesterone acetate, the contraceptive patch, the vaginal ring, the contraceptive implant, and intrauterine devices. Intermenstrual bleeding also may occur if hormonal contraception is not administered as prescribed. Finally, trauma of any origin and other reason, such as excessive exercise or diet, should always be ruled out [4].

6 Menstrual History, Physical Examination, and Laboratory Investigations

Menstrual history should include the age of menarche, the characteristics of the first menstrual period, the general frequency of menstruation, whether menstrual cycles have ever been regular, any associated dysmenorrhea, as well as the timing, duration, and quantity of bleeding during recent menstrual cycles and/or abnormal bleeding episodes. According to Vihko and Apter [12], the role of age at menarche is crucial. Specifically, the patient who is older at menarche is more likely to have a longer time of anovulatory, "irregular" cycles. In girls who describe a change in the menstrual pattern, it is important to ask about other events that coincided with the change, such as stress, weight loss, or an increase in exercise levels. In patients with irregular cycles, maintaining a menstrual calendar is very useful [4]. Patients should be asked regarding any discharge from the breasts. Furthermore, the sexual history should include information regarding contraception and condom use; number of partners; new partners; history of sexually transmitted infections or current symptoms (e.g., vaginal discharge and pelvic pain); and previous pregnancies or terminations [4]. In the medical history, systemic illness, hematologic or renal disease, and current or recent medications should be always taken under consideration, while a history of menstrual disorders in the family may suggest PCOS or other familial endocrine disorders.

The general examination should include vital signs, including pulse and blood pressure levels, measurement of height and weight and calculation of BMI, palpation of the thyroid gland for enlargement, or other abnormalities. Attention should be paid to signs of anemia, as well as any clues of other possible underlying causes. Evaluation for signs of androgen excess includes hirsutism, acne, male pattern balding, and signs of acanthosis nigricans. If the serum prolactin is elevated, the optic fundi should be examined, and visual fields tested to evaluate the possibility of a pituitary tumor. Tanner staging of the breasts and assessment for galactorrhea (bilateral milky nipple discharge) should be conducted, as well as palpation of the abdomen for uterine or ovarian mass. As part of a secondary care approach, an examination of the external genitalia should be carried out whenever indicated. It is also important to look for nonuterine sources of bleeding (e.g., perineal trauma, vulvar lesions, and signs of sexually transmitted infections). Girls, who have signs of perineal trauma, should be questioned privately regarding sexual abuse. When indicated, a speculum examination should be performed in order to rule out the possibility of bleeding ectropion. A bimanual examination should be performed to assess for ovarian or uterine masses and signs of pelvic inflammatory disease. If the history or symptoms suggest pelvic infection, microbiological specimens with a Q tip should be collected from the cervix and vagina. All girls who are sexually active should have a Pap smear and/or HPV DNA test, as per the national cervical screening policy. Finally, evidence of easy bruising or oozing gums should be evaluated for a bleeding disorder [4, 19, 20].

The very first laboratory investigations should include the following: a urine pregnancy test and/or quantitative serum β-HCG and a complete blood cell count with platelet count. A pelvic ultrasound may be very helpful to the diagnosis. According to Brown [21], in cases of severe bleeding or when an underlying bleeding disorder is suspected, the following can be ordered: prothrombin time and partial thromboplastin time, bleeding time and platelet aggregation, von Willebrand panel (must be done prior to initiating hormonal therapy), and factor levels and activity (depending on family history and ethnicity). On the other hand, if an endocrine disorder is suspected, the following laboratory investigations should be made: thyroid-stimulating hormone for screening of thyroid disorders, prolactin (levels

>100 ng/mL suggest a possible pituitary adenoma), total and free testosterone (usually elevated in polycystic ovarian syndrome), dehydroepiandrosterone sulfate to assess for adrenal tumors, luteinizing and follicle-stimulating hormone (may aid in the evaluation of pituitary or ovarian function), sex hormone-binding globulin, fasting lipid profile, fasting plasma glucose level, 17 a-hydroxyprogesterone (elevated in late-onset congenital adrenal hyperplasia), fasting insulin level, and, if indicated, urinary free cortisol, to rule out Cushing's syndrome. If day 3 is not reproducible because of the pattern of bleeding, FSH may be obtained at any time during the cycle. However, the concentration may not be at its nadir, and repeat testing may be necessary to assess the accuracy of the result. In those with raised FSH, karyotype should be carried out. Finally for patients in whom an infectious etiology is suspected, a wet mount of discharge, if bleeding is not severe and a urine nucleic amplification test for gonorrhea and chlamydia should be taken. Pelvic ultrasound is indicated in all women, and transabdominal ultrasound is less sensitive and specific than transvaginal ultrasound but, however, with optimum conditions may still be helpful. Pelvic ultrasound may also indicate uterine structural abnormalities and assist in the diagnosis of PCOS [4, 19, 20].

7 AUB as an Early Sign of PCOS

The menstrual dysfunction usually seen in PCOS reflects chronic anovulation. As a result of this, irregular and infrequent bleeding, which occurs from menarche, is frequently noted. As already mentioned, endometrial proliferation, due to unopposed chronic estrogen secretion, leads to irregular bleeding. There is a connection between irregular menses and anovulation, which is related to the persistence of estrogen production arising primarily from extraglandular conversion of androgens to estrogens. Adolescents with anovulation, which persists more than 2 years, are at greater risk of being diagnosed with PCOS in the near future. It would be no exaggeration to say that the varied menstrual patterns suggest a broad spectrum of phenotypic expression in women with PCOS [21–23].

It is important that 50% of adolescents diagnosed with physiological anovulation have an increase in LH levels and pulse frequency similar to PCOS girls. Lots of efforts have been made to study young adolescents, with irregular bleeding and without hirsutism. 35–63% of these adolescents with persistent anovulation more than 2 years after menarche had increased levels of LH, accompanied by increased pulse frequency and amplitude, together with desynchronization of the circadian profile [14]. Girls with menstrual irregularities and adolescents with normal LH concentrations had similar LH secretion, even though hirsutism was not present in individuals with high LH levels; androgen concentrations were significantly increased, compared with aged-matched normal ovulatory girls [24]. Thus adolescents with menstrual irregularities without hirsutism and elevated serum LH levels might be at increased risk for PCOS. Although the girls who took part in these studies were non-obese, gonadotropin secretion has been found equivalent between obese girls with oligomenorrhea and no clinical or biochemical evidence of hyperandrogenism and obese girls with adolescent PCOS [25]. Increased episodic LH release in non-obese, non-hirsute adolescents with irregular menses or oligomenorrhea has been noted with androgen levels and free androgen index twofold lower than those in the PCOS girls [14].

Additionally, in normal puberty, insulin resistance and compensatory hyperinsulinemia, as a result of pubertal increase in GH production, are usually observed. The insulin resistance of puberty is like that of PCOS in its degree and in its tissue selectivity [16, 26]. Even though insulin together with gonadotropins stimulates ovarian androgen excess, it may contribute to anovulation independently of androgen hypersecretion and explain some AUB cases [27]. It is not yet tested, whether or not this physiological insulin resistance accounts for physiological postmenarchal anovulation.

Furthermore, during the abovementioned anovulation and AUB cases, the ovarian anatomy is very similar with that seen in PCOS. As well known, the normal adolescent ovary histologically resembles a polycystic ovary [28]. The higher number of follicles during menarche, in combination with gonadotropin stimulation, results to greater antral follicles and therefore greater ovarian size [29]. Ultrasounds that have been done in otherwise healthy perimenarchal adolescents have shown multifollicular ovaries, defined as six to ten follicles with a diameter between 4 and 10 mm, but without increase of ovarian stroma [30]. Nearly 8% of asymptomatic postmenarchal adolescents with a polycystic-size ovary were found to have subclinical PCOS, and about half (42%) have a subclinical PCOS type of ovarian dysfunction. Even though these girls didn't have hyperandrogenemia during menarche, they presented with excessive production of 17-OH-PROG in response to GnRH agonist stimulation [28]. So, the syndrome is often perimenarchal in onset presenting similarities with the normal changes of puberty, such as increased ovarian and adrenal steroidogenesis, hyperpulsatile gonadotropin secretion, and menstrual irregularity, including AUB, hyperinsulinemia, and insulin resistance [31, 32].

As already mentioned, menstrual dysfunction and AUB are features of PCOS, which can be observed from menarche. Consistent with this are the results from a large study of patients diagnosed with PCOS by different criteria, in which 75–85% of PCOS girls had clinically evident of menstrual dysfunction sometime during their lifetime [33–35], while in a prospective study of PCOS patients diagnosed among 400 unselected women of the general population, nearly 60% presented with menstrual dysfunction [36]. It is of great importance that women diagnosed with PCOS had more hospitalizations for treatment of gynecological condition, with a higher rate of menstrual problems including excessive, irregular menstruation that also occurred at an earlier age [37]. Furthermore, in another study, which tried to estimate the annual cost in millions of US dollars for menstrual dysfunction or AUB in PCOS, it was found that these conditions represent approximately one third of the overall costs estimated for all admissions due to PCOS. Another important characteristic that was found in this study was that girls with a history of admission diagnosis of excessive menstrual bleeding had four times increased incidence of PCOS in the future [38]. In a cohort study of 136 adolescents by Nair et al. [39], with confirmed menstrual irregularity at menarche, 51.5% continued to have menstrual irregularity, and 36% were diagnosed with PCOS using the Rotterdam criteria at 2 years of follow-up. In another recent study, two thirds of adolescents (66%) who presented with AUB after menarche were diagnosed with PCOS at some time during follow-up, with time of PCOS diagnosis after AUB admission being 2.47 ± 0.78 years [20]. In these adolescents statistically significant differences were noticed in BMI, gonadotropin levels, LH/FSH ratio, as well as in free androgen index and ovarian volume between time of AUB after menarche and diagnosis of PCOS later in their life [20].

8 Management

The management of AUB is based on the underlying etiology and the severity of the bleeding. The prevention of complications, such as anemia, as well as the reestablishment of regular cyclical bleeding, is primarily the goal of controlling AUB. In the case of an underlying systemic, endocrine, or bleeding, patients may require referral to appropriate specialists for further evaluation and management. Several treatment options can be used in the management of AUB such as anti-fibrinolytic tranexamic acid, non-steroidal anti-inflammatory drugs (NSAIDs), combined oral contraception pill (COCs), progestogen, danazol, GnRH analogues, and levonorgestrel-releasing intrauterine system (LNG IUS) device. The most common used during adolescence are COCs and progestogens mainly per os.

The management of AUB in patients with no other etiology will in part be directed by the amount of flow, the degree of associated anemia, as well as patient and family comfort with different treatment modalities [4, 20]. Patients can be divided into four (4) major categories [23]:

- Light to moderate flow; hemoglobin >12 g/dL
  The physician should reassure these patients. An iron supplement can be given, while a nonsteroidal anti-inflammatory drug may help to decrease flow. It is important to re-evaluate patient in 3 months or sooner if bleeding persists or becomes more severe.
- Moderate flow; hemoglobin 10–12 g/dL
  Oral contraceptive pills (OCPs) should be used (e.g., monophasic with 30–35 µg of ethinyl estradiol). One pill twice daily for 1–5 days, until the bleeding stops and once the bleeding stops, OCPs should be continued with a new pack, with one pill daily, for 3–6 months. Iron supplementation for 6 months can be useful, in order to replenish iron stores, while nonsteroidal anti-inflammatory drugs may also be helpful.
- Heavy flow; hemoglobin 8–10 g/dL; hemodynamically stable
  Physician may be able to manage the patient as under "moderate flow" if the family can assist with the management plan and follow-up. If bleeding persists, OCPs should be increased to 3 or 4 times a day for a few days until the bleeding

slows and then two per day and then one pill daily; patient may require an anti-emetic prior to each pill to help prevent nausea. The patient should be followed closely. Once bleeding stops, OCPs should be continued for 6 months.

– Heavy flow; hemoglobin <7 g/dL or if hemodynamically unstable
Patient should be admitted to the hospital. It is important to be considered the possibility of blood transfusion, depending on degree and persistence of bleeding, as well as the severity of hemodynamic instability. Monophasic OCPs should be administered every 6 h until bleeding slows. Then physician should taper administration of pills to one pill a day over the next 7 days (e.g., one pill every 6 h for 2 days, then every 8 h for 2 days, every 12 h for 2 days, then once daily). Antiemetic agents likely will be needed. If bleeding still persists, dilation and curettage should be considered.

In the case of contraindication to estrogens, progesterone, 10 mg once daily for 5–10 days, may be effective for light to moderate flow. Patients also may be cycled monthly on a progesterone-only regimen. Depot medroxyprogesterone acetate, 150 mg intramuscularly every 3 months, or levonorgestrel-releasing intrauterine system device (which lasts for 5 years) can also be used. However the above methods are often associated with irregular bleeding and spotting [23].

9   Discussion

Menstrual disorders and AUB are very common in adolescence. Most of these cases are anovulatory, due to HPO axis immaturity, and the time frame required for maturity of the axis varies between each adolescent. Most of the studies agree that the majority of adolescents have established normal menstrual cycles after the second gynecologic year, while girls with menarche after 13 years old may need 4–5 years to establish 50% ovulatory cycles [12]. Chronic anovulation, unopposed estrogens, and irregular bleeding are linked together, and this can explain why AUB may be the first sign of PCOS later in life. Studies have shown that adolescents with physiological anovulation, which persists more than 2 years, are in greater risk of diagnosed with PCOS in the near future [22, 23]. Furthermore, studies have shown that girls diagnosed with PCOS have a higher rate of menstrual problems including AUB, which occurred at an earlier age [37], while menstrual irregularities and AUB, early after menarche, represent about one third of costs for PCOS [38]. These adolescents are estimated to have a fourfold increased incidence of PCOS in the future [39]. All these findings enhance the correlation between AUB and PCOS. Recently, another study that strengthens this hypothesis was published, in which 66% of postmenarchal girls, who presented with AUB, were diagnosed with PCOS later during follow-up [20]. Therefore, specialized doctors should be alerted when dealing with AUB cases, due to the connection that seems to be appeared, between AUB early after menarche and PCOS later in life.

Another important fact is that the increase in LH levels and pulse frequency in normal anovulatory adolescents after menarche is similar to PCOS girls. Increased

LH levels, pulse frequency, and desynchronization of the circadian profile have been reported in 35–63% of adolescents who still had anovulatory cycles 2 years after menarche [14]. Girls with anovulation and elevated LH levels, without hirsutism, had significantly increased androgen concentrations compared with aged-matched normal ovulatory girls [24]. This finding is corroborated by another study, which showed that girls with AUB early after menarche with a diagnosis of PCOS later in life had statistically significant increased levels of free androgen index (FAI) but no differences in hirsutism or LH levels, when compared with adolescents who presented with AUB after menarche, but were never diagnosed with PCOS until late adolescence [20]. It is generally accepted that LH levels, pulse frequency, and desynchronization of its circadian profile play a crucial role in anovulation and androgen production, despite the absence of clinical hyperandrogenism (hirsutism, acne). Additionally, hyperinsulinemia, as a result of pubertal increase in GH and IGF-1 production and insulin resistance of puberty, resembles that seen in PCOS regarding its degree and its tissue selectivity [16, 26]. Insulin acts in ovaries producing androgens and furthermore contributes to anovulation. So, all these procedures mentioned above, which can expressed clinically as AUB after menarche, may still be at an early stage and not yet reached in degree all these criteria needed for the diagnosis of PCOS. Consistent with this is that several studies have shown that the signs of PCOS start to appear early after menarche and a time interval is required to manifest the syndrome.

It is also important that during menarche many follicles can be observed in ovaries. As a result of gonadotropin stimulation to these follicles, more antral follicles and greater ovarian size are noted in these adolescents [29]. During anovulation and AUB cases early after menarche, the ovarian anatomy is very similar with that seen in PCOS. In a study by Merrill [28], it was shown that 8% of asymptomatic postmenarchal adolescents with a polycystic-sized ovary were found to have subclinical PCOS and 42% have a subclinical PCOS type of ovarian dysfunction. In another study girls with AUB early after menarche, with a diagnosis of PCOS later in life, were found to have greater ovarian volume, when compared with adolescents who presented with AUB after menarche but were never diagnosed with PCOS until late adolescence [20]. The difference was more prominent after 3 years of follow-up, at time of PCOS diagnosis. These studies show that there is a predisposition in ovary morphology for the diagnosis of PCOS later in life. Nevertheless, more studies should be conducted to confirm these results.

10 Conclusion

In conclusion, AUB is a common cause for concern among adolescents and their families, while PCOS remains the most common endocrine disorder during adolescence. AUB cases reflect the immaturity of HPO axis and may be an early symptom of PCOS in some adolescents. A lot of similarities seem to appear between normal changes in puberty and PCOS later in adolescence including increased ovarian and adrenal steroidogenesis, hyperpulsatile gonadotropin secretion, hyperinsulinemia and insulin resistance, anovulation, and therefore menstrual irregularity, including AUB. Persistent chronic anovulation may be expressed in the beginning of adolescence as AUB and still enhances the diagnosis of PCOS later in life. It is very important that girls presenting with AUB should seek help from specialized doctors in pediatric and adolescent gynecology in referral centers and should be carefully evaluated and properly followed up until late adolescence, due to the fact that they are in increased risk to be diagnosed with PCOS. An early intervention may be crucial in future general health and fertility of these adolescents.

References

1. Munro MG, Critchley HO, Broder MS, Fraser IS, FIGO Working Group on Menstrual Disorders. FIGO classification system (PALM-COEIN) for causes of abnormal uterine bleeding in nongravid women of reproductive age. Int J Gynaecol Obstet. 2011;113(1):3–13.
2. Fraser IS, Langham S, Uhl-Hochgraeber K. Health-related quality of life and economic burden of abnormal uterine bleeding. Exp Rev Obstet Gynecol. 2009;4:179–89.
3. Matteson KA, Baker CA, Clark MA, Frick KD. Abnormal uterine bleeding, health status, and usual source of medical care: analyses using the medical expenditures panel survey. J Womens Health (Larchmt). 2013;22:959–65.
4. Deligeoroglou E, Karountzos V, Creatsas G. Abnormal uterine bleeding and dysfunctional uterine bleeding in pediatric and adolescent gynecology. Gynecol Endocrinol. 2013;29(1):74–8.
5. Farquhar C. Introduction and history of polycystic ovary syndrome. In: Kovacs G, Norman R, editors. Polycystic ovary syndrome. 2nd ed. Cambridge, UK: Cambridge University Press; 2007. p. 4–24.
6. Balen A, Conway G, Kaltsas G. Polycystic ovary syndrome: the spectrum of the disorder in 1741 patients. Hum Reprod. 1995;10:2107–11.
7. Fauser B, Tarlatzis B, Rebar R, Legro RS, Balen AH, Lobo R, et al. Consensus on women's health aspects of polycystic ovary syndrome (PCOS): the Amsterdam ESHRE/ASRM-sponsored 3rd PCOS consensus workshop group. Fertil Steril. 2012;97(1):28–38.
8. Carmina E. Diagnosis of polycystic ovary syndrome: from NIH criteria to ESHRE-ASRM guidelines. Minerva Ginecol. 2004;56(1):1–6.
9. Finer LB, Philbin JM. Trends in ages at key reproductive transitions in the United States, 1951–2010. Womens Health Issues. 2014;24:e 271–9.
10. Chumlea WC, Schubert CM, Roche AF, Kulin HE, Lee PA, Himes JH, et al. Age at menarche and racial comparisons in US girls. Pediatrics. 2003;111:110–3.
11. ACOG Committee on Adolescent Health Care. ACOG Committee Opinion no. 349, November 2006: menstruation in girls and adolescents: using the menstrual cycle as a vital sign. Obstet Gynecol. 2006;108(5):1323–8.
12. Apter D, Vihko R. Early menarche, a risk factor for breast cancer, indicates early onset of ovulatory cycles. J Clin Endocrinol Metab. 1983;57(1):82–6.
13. Apter D, Vihko R. Serum pregnenolone, progesterone, 17-hydroxyprogesterone, testosterone, and 5α-dihydrotestosterone during female puberty. J Clin Endocrinol Metab. 1977;45:1039–48.
14. Venturoli S, Porcu E, Fabbri R, Magrini O, Gammi L, Paradisi R, et al. Longitudinal evaluation of the different gonadotropin pulsatile patterns in anovulatory cycles of young girls. J Clin Endocrinol Metab. 1992;74:836–41.
15. Southam A, Richart E. The prognosis for adolescents with menstrual abnormalities. Am J Obstet Gynecol. 1966;94:637.
16. Amiel SA, Caprio S, Sherwin RS, Plewe G, HaymondMW TWV. Insulin resistance of puberty: a defect restricted to peripheral glucose metabolism. J Clin Endocrinol Metab. 1991;72:277–82.

17. Vaginal CG, Bleedings U. In: Creatsas GK, editor. Obstetrics and gynecology of young age. 1st ed. Athens: P. X Paschalidis; 2001. p. 273–6.
18. Deligeoroglou E, Karountzos V. Abnormal uterine bleeding including coagulopathies and other menstrual disorders. Best Pract Res Clin Obstet Gynaecol. 2018 Apr;48:51–61.
19. Deligeoroglou E. Dysfunctional uterine bleeding. Ann N Y Acad Sci. 1997;816:158–64.
20. Deligeoroglou EK, Creatsas GK. Dysfunctional uterine bleeding as an early sign of polycystic ovary syndrome during adolescence. Minerva Ginecol. 2015;67(4):375–81.
21. Livingstone M, Fraser IS. Mechanisms of abnormal uterine bleeding. Hum Reprod Update. 2002;8:60–7.
22. World Health Organization task force on adolescent reproductive health. World Health Organization multicenter study on menstrual and ovulatory patterns in adolescent girls. II. Longitudinal study of menstrual patterns in the early postmenarcheal period, duration of bleeding episodes and menstrual cycles. J Adolesc Health Care. 1986;7(4):236–44.
23. Hickey M, Balen A. Menstrual disorders in adolescence: investigation and management. Hum Reprod Update. 2003;9:493–504.
24. Porcu E, Venturoli S, Magrini O, Bolzani R, Gabbi D, Paradisi R, et al. Circadian variations of luteinizing hormone can have two different profiles in adolescent anovulation. J Clin Endocrinol Metab. 1987;65:488–93.
25. Yoo RY, Dewan A, Basu R, Newfield R, Gottschalk M, Chang RJ. Increased luteinizing hormone pulse frequency in obese oligomenorrheic girls with no evidence of hyperandrogenism. Fertil Steril. 2006;85:1049–56.
26. Moran A, Jacobs DR Jr, Steinberger J, Hong CP, Prineas R, Luepker R, et al. Insulin resistance during puberty: results from clamp studies in 357 children. Diabetes. 1999;48:2039–44.
27. Franks S. Controversy in clinical endocrinology: diagnosis of polycystic ovarian syndrome: in defense of the Rotterdam criteria. J Clin Endocrinol Metab. 2006;91:786–9.
28. Merrill JA. The morphology of the prepubertal ovary: relationship to the polycystic ovary syndrome. South Med J. 1963;56:225–31.
29. Mortensen M, Rosenfield R, Littlejohn E. Functional significance of polycystic-size ovaries in healthy adolescents. J Clin Enocrinol Metab. 2006;91:3786–90.
30. Brook C, Jacobs H, StanhopeR. Polycystic ovaries in childhood. Br Med J. 1988;296:878.
31. Poretsky L. Polycystic ovary syndrome: increased or preserved ovarian sensitivity to insulin? J Clin Endocrinol Metab. 2006;91:2859–60.
32. Leibel NI, Baumann EE, Kocherginsky M, Rosenfield RL. Relationship of adolescent polycystic ovary syndrome to parental metabolic syndrome. J Clin Endocrinol Metab. 2006;91:1275–83.
33. Azziz R, Sanchez LA, Knochenhauer ES, Moran C, Lazenby J, Stephens KC, et al. Androgen excess in women: experience with over 1000 consecutive patients. J Clin Endocrinol Metab. 2004;89:453–62.
34. Goldzieher JW, Axelrod LR. Clinical and biochemical features of polycystic ovarian disease. Fertil Steril. 1963;14:631–53.
35. Conway GS, Honour JW, Jacobs HS. Heterogeneity of the polycystic ovary syndrome: clinical, endocrine and ultrasound features in 556 patients. Clin Endocrinol. 1989;30:459–70.
36. Azziz R, Woods KS, Reyna R, Key TJ, Knochenhauer ES, Yildiz BO. The prevalence and features of the polycystic ovary syndrome in an unselected population. J Clin Endocrinol Metab. 2004;89:2745–9.
37. Hart R, Doherty DA. The potential implications of a PCOS diagnosis on a woman's long-term health using data linkage. J Clin Endocrinol Metab. 2015;100(3):911–9.
38. Azziz R, Marin C, Hoq L, Badamgarav E, Song P. Health care-related economic burden of the polycystic ovary syndrome during the reproductive life span. J Clin Endocrinol Metab. 2005;90(8):4650–8.
39. Nair MK, Pappachan P, Balakrishnan S, Leena ML, George B, Russell PS. Menstrual irregularity and poly cystic ovarian syndrome among adolescent girls—a 2 year follow-up study. Indian J Pediatr. 2012;79(Suppl 1):S69–73.

How to Identify Patients with von Willebrand's Disease and Other Coagulation Disorders

Gabriele Susanne Merki-Feld

1 Introduction

Abnormal uterine bleeding (AUB) is a frequently reported symptom, especially during adolescence and the late reproductive years. According to the FIGO classification 2018, AUB comprises abnormalities in frequency, duration, regularity, and volume of the menstrual bleeding [1]. Heavy menstrual bleeding (HMB) is defined as a flow volume that interferes with the woman's quality of life and insofar depends on the patient's subjective perception and does not imply that there is a causative medical condition. It may however cause iron deficiency on the long term and reduce well-being and capacity. Insofar, discrimination between a normal and a pathologic bleeding tendency is relevant [2]. A more detailed history on the number of sanitary pads used together with a bleeding chart might help to better assess the blood loss. Women with a high blood loss might also report the loss of clots. Earlier studies report a mean blood loss of 43.4 mL for a normal menstrual bleeding. However, 19% of all women will have a loss of more than 60 mL and 11% more than 80 mL [3, 4]. A blood loss of >60 mL is significantly associated with the development of anemia. The patient history in a woman with HMB should also include questions about medical conditions and medications. In particular treatment with anticoagulants should be excluded.

G. S. Merki-Feld (✉)
Clinic for Reproductive Medicine, University Hospital Zürich, Zürich, Switzerland
e-mail: gabriele.merki@usz.ch

© The Author(s), under exclusive license to Springer Nature Switzerland AG 2024

A. R. Genazzani et al. (eds.), *Menstrual Bleeding and Pain Disorders from Adolescence to Menopause*, ISGE Series,
https://doi.org/10.1007/978-3-031-55300-4_5

2 Organic and Other Not Hematologic Causes of HMB

Organic causes of HMB include leiomyoma, polyps, adenomyosis, malignancies, and endometrial hyperplasia. They are described in detail in the FIGO classification 2018 [1]. Mostly a gynecologic check with ultrasound can confirm or exclude such a condition. In adolescents and during perimenopause, ovulatory dysfunction is a frequent underlying reason for HMB. Women treated with anticoagulant medicines also tend to have prolonged bleeding and heavier flow.

3 Heavy Menstrual Bleeding in Patients with Von Willebrand Disease (VWD)

Von Willebrand factor (VWF) is a multimeric protein with two main hemostatic functions:

1. In primary hemostasis at the site of injured vessel walls, it facilitates platelet adhesion to subendothelial structures and supports platelet aggregation and thrombus formation.
2. As part of secondary hemostasis, VWF acts as a carrier protein for coagulation factor VIII (FVIII), stabilizing and protecting FVIII procoagulant activity.

Von Willebrand disease (VWD), a deficiency in VWF, is the most common inherited bleeding disorder, yet diagnosis and management remain challenging. The prevalence is around 16% among the Caucasian population (Table 1). Although 74–92% of affected women experience HMB, mild forms of this coagulation disorders can easily be overlooked, as 40% of all women with HMB would think that their bleedings are normal [5]. Furthermore physicians have to be aware that 25% of women with normal blood loss will report that their bleeding is too heavy [6]. Early diagnosis of a coagulation disorder is relevant especially in females, to prevent complications during deliveries, but also in the case of injuries or surgery. Awareness for this condition needs to be raised, as today still only a subset of women with HMB are screened for a coagulopathy. The understanding that bleeding histories are very subjective leads to several attempts to standardize diagnostic criteria and methods that collect data to determine the presence and the severity of bleeding symptoms. The key question is which patient with HMB should be screened for a disorder of

Table 1 Prevalence of bleeding disorders in women with menorrhagia

Bleeding disorder	Prevalence
Von Willebrand disease	5–20%
Caucasian population	16%
Platelet dysfunction	<1–47%
Factor XI deficiency	<1–4%
Hemophilia carriage	<1–4%

hemostasis after gynecologic abnormalities have been excluded. Meanwhile hematologic societies developed a reliable, but complex score system [7, 8]. For daily use gynecologists might prefer to work with an easier approach using key questions for a broader specific history (Table 2). For adolescents this has to be taken into account, because they might not yet have experienced deliveries, surgery, or dental procedures. Insofar they might have lower screening scores, but nevertheless suffer from VWD. It is worthwhile to specifically focus on family history here.

4   Which Women with HMB Need Screening for Coagulopathy After Uterine Pathology Has Been Excluded?

Women with coagulation disorders will suffer from HMB often beginning at menarche. The family history for HMB is often positive. They typically experience further symptoms like bruising with minimal trauma, prolonged bleeding from trivial wounds, epistaxis >10 min or requiring medical attention, frequent gum bleeding, heavy bleeding after dental procedures, surgical-related bleeding, gastrointestinal bleeding, and postpartum hemorrhage (Table 2) [1, 8]. They might also have a history of anemia with iron therapy. In-depth history of the bleeding pattern might help to better assess the blood (Table 3). Detailed screening tools with scores have been elaborated to better assess which patients should be referred to a hematologist (Table 2) [7]. For practitioners referring a patient to test for VWD, it is of relevance

Table 2 Clinical symptoms indicating VWD as potential cause of heavy menstrual bleeding

Heavy menstrual bleeding since menarche	
One of the following	Postpartum hemorrhage Surgical-related bleeding Bleeding associated with dental work
Two or more of the following symptoms	Bruising 1–2 times/months Epistaxis 1–2 times/months Frequent gum bleeding Positive family history of bleeding symptoms

Table 3 Key questions to evaluate menstrual blood loss more objective

Number of bleeding days/cycle
Frequency of the cycle
Number of days with heavy bleeding
Number of pads used at the days with heavy bleeding
Loss of blood clots
Time of onset of the heavy bleeding
History of medical conditions
History of medications used: anticoagulants?

that VWF is increased during use of hormonal contraceptives and hormone replacement therapy. It should be discussed with the hematologist if there is a need to interrupt hormone use to get an accurate diagnosis [6].

5   Treatment Options of HMB in Women Without an Organic Cause of the Condition

Treatment of HMB in women will depend on the cause of HMB. If organic causes have been excluded, cyclic hormonal treatment will be an option in women with ovulatory dysfunction (adolescence, perimenopause, other reasons), but also those with coagulopathy, if the symptoms are mild. In VWD patients with more symptoms, pregnancies, and before surgery, collaboration with the hematologist is recommended. Replacement of VWF or desmopressin might be used here.

5.1   Treatment of Women with HMB Only, No Organic Cause, No Coagulation Disorder

1. No need for contraception

   - Cyclic norethisterone 3×5 mg from cycle days 7–28 is more effective than cyclic medroxyprogesterone acetate. The duration of treatment can be adapted and shortened if the blood loss is less intense.
   - Tranexamic acid 4 g from cycle days 1–5.

2. Need for contraception

   - All combined hormonal contraceptives (CHC) reduce the menstrual flow. Progestins like dienogest, desogestrel, and gestoden exert a stronger suppressive effect on the endometrium and are therefore superior in comparison to combinations with ethinylestradiol (EE) and levonorgestrel (LNG). However, the risk for venous thromboembolism is slightly higher for CHC with dienogest and third-generation progestins.
   - Levonorgestrel-releasing device releasing 20 µg LNG is highly effective.
   - Progestin-only contraceptives (POC) can cause prolonged menorrhagia in healthy women. Insofar only some of the available progestin-only contraceptives (POC) can be used in women with HMB. The desogestrel-only pill and the etonogestrel-releasing implant are very low dosed. They frequently cause additional bleeding problems in women with HMB. The 12-weekly injection of depot medroxyprogesterone acetate (DMPA) might also cause menorrhagia during the initial months of use; however this problem can be solved by using a shorter injection interval of 8 or 10 weeks, when

starting the method. The interval between injections can also be adapted according to the bleeding pattern on the long term. The majority of patients will develop amenorrhea with longer duration of use. DMPA is not recommended for use in adolescents, as it has a negative impact on the development of peak bone density.

5.2   Treatment of Women with HMB Only, No Organic Cause, VWD, or Other Coagulation Disorder

1. No need for contraception

   - Tranexamic acid 4 g from cycle days 1–5 might be the first treatment option and is also effective in women with acute bleeding.
   - Cyclic norethisterone 3 × 5 mg from cycle days 7–28. The duration of treatment can be adapted.

2. Need for contraception

   - The same choices of COC and POC, or the LNG 20 μg device can be used, as in other women with HMB.

6   Conclusion

HMB is one leading symptom of VWD in women. HMB however is very subjective and also widespread in patients without VWD. After organic causes have been excluded, an in-depth patient history about the menstrual bleeding and for VWD specific symptoms, using the FIGO criteria, is helpful in the decision, if a patient should be screened for coagulation disease.

References

1. Munro MG, Critchley HOD, Fraser IS, Committee FMD. The two FIGO systems for normal and abnormal uterine bleeding symptoms and classification of causes of abnormal uterine bleeding in the reproductive years: 2018 revisions. Int J Gynaecol Obstet. 2018;143(3):393–408.
2. de Moerloose P, Levrat E, Fontana P, Boehlen F. Diagnosis of mild bleeding disorders. Swiss Med Wkly. 2009;139(23–24):327–32.
3. Hallberg L, Hogdahl AM, Nilsson L, Rybo G. Menstrual blood loss and iron deficiency. Acta Med Scand. 1966;180(5):639–50.
4. Cole S. Menstrual blood loss and haematological indices. J Reprod Fertil. 1971;27(1):158.
5. Committee on Adolescent Health Care, Committee on Gynecologic Practice. Committee Opinion No. 580: von Willebrand disease in women. Obstet Gynecol. 2013;122(6):1368–73.

6. Tosetto A, Rodeghiero F, Castaman G, Goodeve A, Federici AB, Batlle J, et al. A quantitative analysis of bleeding symptoms in type 1 von Willebrand disease: results from a multicenter European study (MCMDM-1 VWD). J Thromb Haemost. 2006;4(4):766–73.
7. Pathare A, Al Omrani S, Al Hajri F, Al Obaidani N, Al Balushi B, Al Falahi K. Bleeding score in type 1 von Willebrand disease patients using the ISTH-BAT questionnaire. Int J Lab Hematol. 2018;40(2):175–80.
8. Tosetto A, Castaman G, Rodeghiero F. Assessing bleeding in von Willebrand disease with bleeding score. Blood Rev. 2007;21(2):89–97.

Anovulatory Syndrome

Veronica Tomatis, Elisa Semprini, Christian Battipaglia, Tabatha Petrillo, and Alessandro D. Genazzani

1 Introduction

Woman biology is a complex system ruled by various endocrine axes: every axis has its own role, but they still manage to work together effectively [1]. The most notable feature of the female reproductive system is the absence of a steady state, and its optimal performance is founded on the equilibrium of various elements of each axis (i.e., the hypothalamus, the pituitary, and the ovary) with the other hormonal axes regulated in concert by distinct cell nuclei in the pituitary gland (gonadotropic, thyrotropic, lactotrophs, somatotropic, and corticotropic cells).

Our biological system is dynamic and interactive, based on genetic and epigenetic relationships and conditioned by environmental factors in most cases. Whenever the menstrual cyclicity is altered, a menstrual and ovulatory impairment occurs. Many adaptations in reproductive ability are primarily linked to a modification of those fine mechanisms that control ovulation induction. It is well known that gonadotropin secretion is under the modulation of a number of steroids (i.e., estrogen, androgens, cortisol, etc.) as well as of neuropeptides (i.e., opioids, catecholamines, neuropeptides) that act directly on GnRH or kisspeptin neurons as well as on gonadotrope cells (Fig. 1).

The GnRH neurons' secretory activity and the receptor expression are in charge of the reproductive system, modulated by positive and negative factors. The biggest driving force of GnRH discharge is kisspeptin, whose receptors are expressed on GnRH neurons [2, 3]. As for many neuroendocrine systems, kisspeptin is very sensitive to signal coming from the periphery—mainly metabolic signals such as

V. Tomatis · E. Semprini · C. Battipaglia · T. Petrillo · A. D. Genazzani (✉)
Department of Obstetrics and Gynecology, Gynecological Endocrinology Center,
University of Modena and Reggio Emilia, Modena, Italy
e-mail: algen@unimo.it

A. R. Genazzani et al. (eds.), *Menstrual Bleeding and Pain Disorders from Adolescence to Menopause*, ISGE Series,
https://doi.org/10.1007/978-3-031-55300-4_6

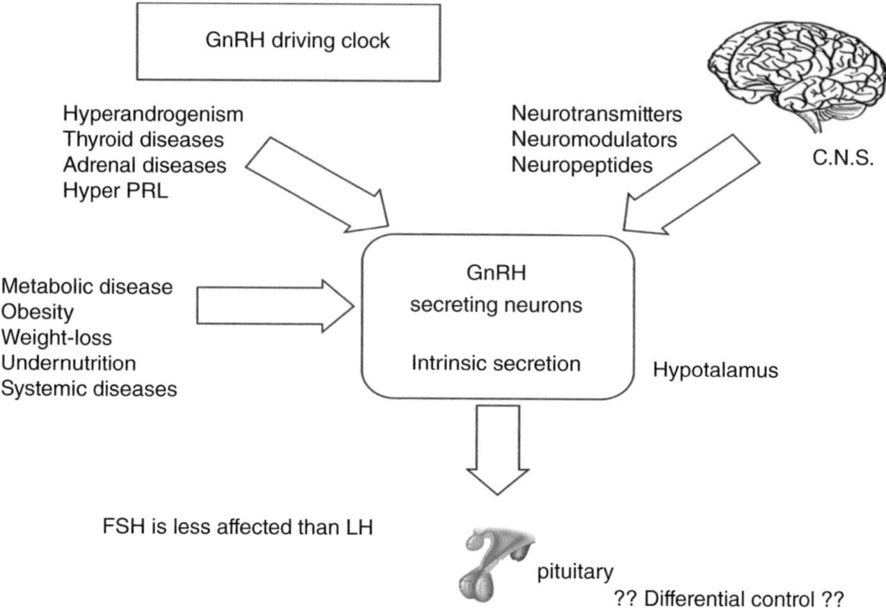

Fig. 1 The whole reproductive system depends on GnRH neurons' secretory activity and on receptor expression, which are modulated by positive and negative factors so as to activate or impair their functions. FSH seems to be less affected than LH by all such modulatory system

ghrelin, cholecystokinin, leptin, and insulin [4]—and it is greatly affected by changes coming from the gastro-intestinal tract [5].

All these modulators of kisspeptin and GnRH release indirectly affect the release of gonadotropins. Stressful situations such as psychological, physical, or metabolic stressors, together with weight fluctuations, can induce an impaired neuroendocrine function at the hypothalamic level through the impaired production of amines, beta-endorphin, and serotonin [6]. All of them can interfere in the regulation of GnRH, thus influencing the reproductive capacity overall [7].

Gonadal steroids also play an important role in the modulation of the GnRH-induced gonadotropin secretion, since estrogen and androgens are able to greatly interfere in the amount of LH released from the pituitary through the feedback control system [8]. The role exerted by estrogen has been recently demonstrated in some pathological conditions since estriol administration was able to induce a greater response of gonadotrope cells to both exogenous and endogenous GnRH stimulation [9, 10].

In addition, impairments of the main endocrine axes that regulate our biology (thyroid, adrenal, and prolactin axis) have been demonstrated to cause changes in the reproductive ability and in the menstrual cyclicity.

The endocrine factors that trigger the chronic anovulation and disrupt the control system of the reproductive axis are hyperandrogenic states, of adrenal or ovarian origin, hypo- or hyperthyroidism, and hyperprolactinemia, but also peripheral signals, in particular the balance of metabolism and stress, are extremely important to interfere with the control of reproduction [1, 11].

Peripheral endocrine disorders create abnormal modulation from peripheral systems and glands. In case these events are additional to central dysfunction, all this generates abnormal control of the hypothalamus, pituitary, and ovary, developing chronic anovulation. Chronic anovulation occurs as consequence of stress, altered BMI, hyperandrogenic signs, and amenorrhea or oligomenorrhea.

2 Hypothalamic Amenorrhea

When no endocrine factor is recognized, a hypothalamic blockade has to be suspected and investigated. Such kind of amenorrhea is called hypothalamic, and it is associated with metabolic, physical, or psychological stress.

Affective disorders (neuroticism, somatization, anxiety) are often associated to a psychological stressor and heavy negative event, and this leads to the disruption of the hypothalamus-pituitary activity, and as a consequence, there is an abnormal and, later, the block of the ovarian function [12].

These physical, psychological, and metabolic conditions are identified as "stressors" and negatively affect GnRH release and the reproductive axis, activating or inhibiting hypothalamic and/or extra-hypothalamic areas in the brain as well as acting in the periphery (Fig. 2). Each of these signals may become stressor agents and stimulate adaptive responses. Every occurring negative hypothalamic response is

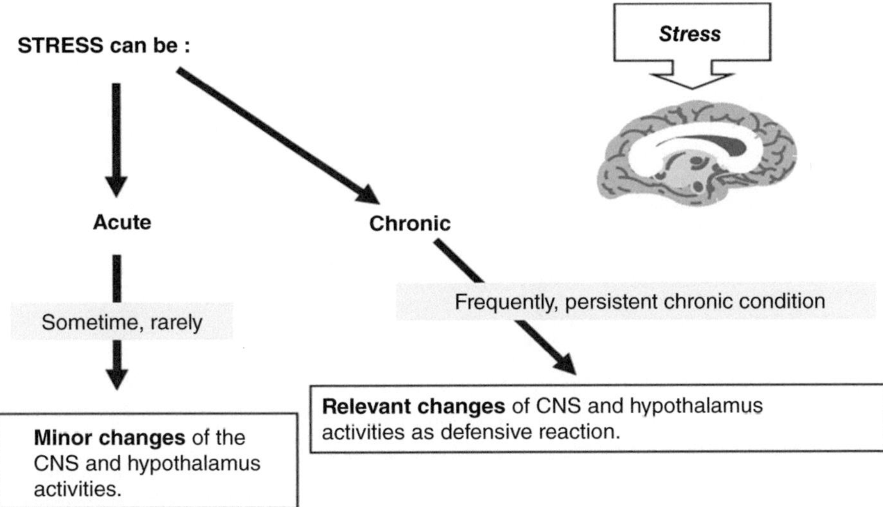

Fig. 2 Stress-induced neuroendocrine malfunction occurs only when such stressors act in a chronic manner

defensive. In human females an adaptive mechanism is represented by the reduction of reproductive axis activity, stopping a function considered not essential to survive.

Therefore anytime every stressor (dieting, sport, training, or psychological stressors) hits the human being, the adaptive response induced by biological systems and deeply linked to our evolutionary facts reacts as if induced by the attack of a wild animal or by lack of food and/or by strenuous fatigue due to a migration.

Since corticotropin-releasing hormone (CRF) is the specific hypothalamic stimulating factor for ACTH, stress elevation of ACTH is anticipated by the elevation of CRF stimulation (Fig. 3). The evidence of a central site of action for CRF in blocking GnRH-induced LH release is demonstrated by the fact that CRF antagonists reverse the stress-induced LH decrease in rats [13]. CRF elevation as adaptive response to stress is also responsible for the increase of central ß-endorphin (ßEP) release. This last is probably the most important peptide of the endogenous opioid peptide family, and it is a potent inhibitor of GnRH-LH secretion. Because of this evidence, a connection is suggested between the activation of the hypothalamus-pituitary-adrenal (HPA) axis and the stress inhibition of the hypothalamus-pituitary-gonadal (HPG) axis [14]. This mechanism is mediated by the activation of several stimulating factors like thyrotropin-releasing hormone, vasoactive intestinal

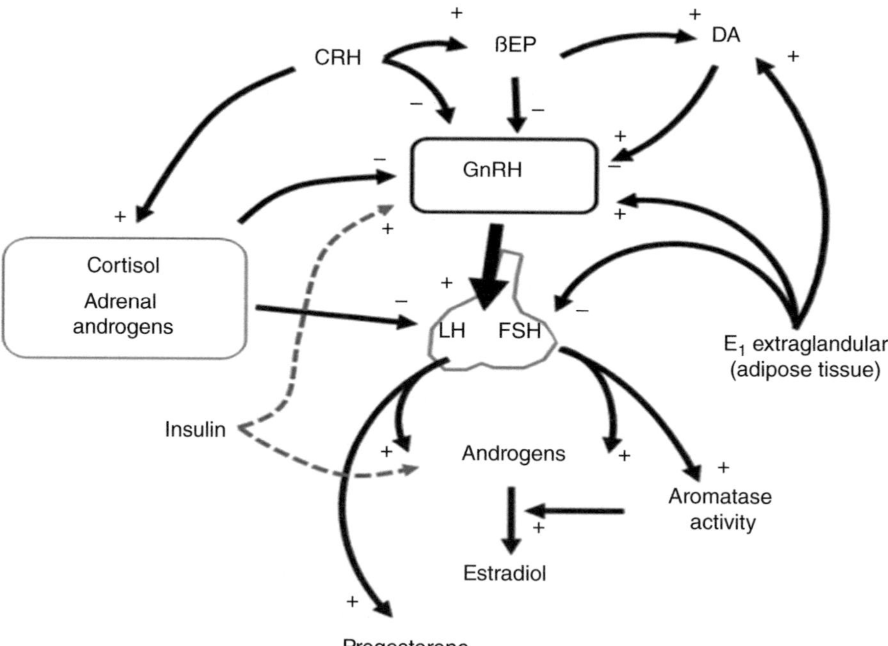

Fig. 3 GnRH-secreting neurons undergo to positive and negative modulations. Stress, through CRH activation, determines a slowing down of GnRH secretion together with opioid peptides (β-endorphin, BEP). Insulin, especially in hyperinsulinemic PCOS patients, stimulates ovarian androgen synthesis and LH release, thus improving the ovarian impairment. *DA* dopamine, *CRH* corticotropin-releasing hormone, *E1* estrone, *βEP* beta endorphin

peptide, and oxytocin or by the failure of the dopaminergic control. Finally the result of stress-related hormone responses is a negative effect both on gonadotropin secretion and on gonadal steroid biosynthesis.

It is of interest to observe that in hypothalamic amenorrhea, LH seems to be the more sensitive to the hypothalamus functional impairment, since only LH plasma levels are significantly reduced [15–17]. The meaning of such biological event can be easily explained by the fact that it is the LH ovulatory surge that triggers ovulation. No LH, no ovulation.

Stress responses induced by dieting or excessive energy expense, such as in athletes, triggers similar neuropeptides with the addition of the negative modulation induced by the lack of energy availability (i.e., reduced fat mass, feeding using low caloric diet). In such conditions, it has been reported that acetyl-L-carnitine (ALC) administration is effective in inducing the recovery of the endogenous as well as the exogenous GnRH-induced LH secretion [18].

The fact that stress and anxiety both stimulate the secretion of corticotropin-releasing factor (CRF) and modulate GABAergic neurons suggests a possible functional interaction between these two systems. Indeed, GABAergic or benzodiazepine receptor-mediated mechanisms inhibit CRF release [19].

It is well known that gonadal steroids (i.e., estrogens and progesterone) play a relevant role on the modulation of the hypothalamus and pituitary functions. Recently, our group demonstrated that the daily administration of estriol at low dosage of 2 mg/day for 8 weeks was effective in increasing both LH plasma levels and the amplitude of LH pulses [10]. In addition, estriol administration determined also a significant increase of LH response to the GnRH exogenous infusion [10]. Also using hyperlow doses of estradiol, as low as 1 µg, confirms these results. This hyperlow estrogenic treatment is probably able to induce an effect at the hypothalamic and pituitary level similar to estriol administration [8], which is an increased sensitivity to GnRH and a higher expression of GnRH receptors, thus permitting the increase of LH synthesis and secretion.

3 Weight and Reproduction

A specific correlation exists between loss of weight and amenorrhea [20, 21], and the loss of weight below a critical point and the reduced ratio between fat and muscular masses lead to the loss of menstrual cyclicity. Secondly, but important to frame the patient, psychological stressors may also have an impact on food intake.

Obesity and malnutrition, the two opposite aspects of alterations of metabolism, are particularly critical because they block the reproductive system, inducing impaired hypothalamic activity aspects as a defensive mechanism to avoid pregnancy and adverse pregnancy-induced side effects.

In fact reduced or increased BMI is responsible for impaired reproductive function through the reduced or excessive release of the specific neuroendocrine modulators that act on the kisspeptin-GnRH neurons and impair the LH secretory pattern and reproduction [4].

Moreover a lack or excess of nutrients creates specific impaired neuroendocrine responses to reduce or block follicle recruitment and then reproduction [6, 22–24]. In particular, though adipose tissue is not a gland, it manages the synthesis of hormones like an endocrine organ. It is clear that a situation of overweight up to obesity can change not only the adiponectins and leptin produced, but also the steroids milieu. Any excess of these substances is able to interfere in the hypothalamic functions, together with insulin acting on kisspeptin neurons, thus affecting GnRH neurons' activity [25, 26].

In addition, adipocytes produce androstenedione, estrone, and estriol and can absorb therapeutically administered steroids [23]. Such estrogen and progestogen uptake permits their release back into circulation in variable moments and amounts later, causing severe fluctuations of plasma concentrations [27]. It is therefore very important to explain to patients how relevant is to follow healthy eating attitude, in order to limit the deposition of adipose tissue and to have an optimal body weight.

A clear correlation exists between the incidence of reproductive function and the percentage of body weight loss [28, 29]. In fact, the suppression of the central drives to the HPG axis in undernutrition takes place only with a significant loss of body fat [29, 30].

4 Hyperandrogenism

Androgens are essential for the function of the cerebral cortex, because they increase critical abilities, adaptation, and sexuality [31]. In fact, the ovary production of androgens is reduced during menopause: this causes the gradual decrease in these abilities, in particular libido and sexuality. However, the adrenal gland decreases its activity in a chronologically similar way both in men and women. Furthermore, folliculogenesis, in mice, does not operate properly in the absence of the androgen signal [32, 33].

On the other hand, follicle development is impaired when there is an excess of androgens. Hyperandrogenism can also be triggered by a chronic situation of stress and might generate a series of consequences. This happens in polycystic ovary syndrome (PCOS) that shows both hyperandrogenism and anovulation and, often, infertility [32].

Cortisol can modulate the reproductive axis with central actions, affecting the synthesis of gonadotropins and also directly on the ovary, interfering with the synthesis and release of estrogen and of progesterone during the luteal phase.

Stressful situations cause cortisol elevation, and this slows down the reproductive axis: when stress becomes chronic, menstrual disorders occur more frequently, even up to amenorrhea [34].

In fact, high levels of glucocorticoids inhibit GnRH neurons' activity, thus affecting gonadotrope cells and gonadal function [35]. CRH infusion during the midluteal phase reduces plasma LH and FSH levels, while their concentrations return to normal levels as soon as CRH infusion is stopped. Interestingly, CRH infusion did not alter the gonadotropin response to GnRH bolus, thus confirming that CRH acts at the hypothalamic level [36]. The key point is a restraint action on aromatase that is sensitive to alterations such as an excess of androgens, prolactin, and hyperinsulinemia; by modulating the activity of aromatase, the androgen levels change accordingly [23].

Additionally, stress through adrenal gland hyperactivation increases cortisol and consequentially gluconeogenesis, thus favoring obesity and hyperandrogenism; this leads to a growing endocrine impairment and might favor greater cardiovascular risk, the primary cause of death in women over 50. Moreover, the excess of cortisol interferes with insulin and growth factors promoting mechanisms that predispose one to a greater oncological risk [37, 38].

5 Polycystic Ovary Syndrome (PCOS)

In PCOS, hyperandrogenism is the key element that induces anovulation [39]. Too many androgens limit the ovarian function, making ovaries assume the classic PCO morphology. If we assume that a PCO ovary is the only cause of the hyperandrogenic state, we might miss the real cause of anovulation. Another element to consider is hyperinsulinemia, very frequent in obese PCOS: insulin stimulates GnRH release and consequently gonadotropin secretion that stimulate the production of ovarian steroids (especially androstenedione) with inhibitory action on aromatase. This results in an excess of androgens not converted to estrogen. Insulin also inhibits sex hormone-binding globulin (SHBG) with an increase in free androgens (Fig. 1). It is clear that hyperinsulinemia represents a fundamental issue in the case of PCOS, since it favors the condition of hyperandrogenism with greater amounts of free plasma androgens [40] and specific negative effects on liver function [25, 41].

PCOS women might be hyperandrogenic, with the contribution of the adrenal gland even though it does not have an impaired adrenal function: the PCOS clinical condition is often characterized by an increased psychological stress that triggers the adrenal activity [42]. PCOS patients also may show an increase in cortisol and 17-OHP plasma levels [43].

These women had a more activated adrenal gland in baseline conditions, with no abnormal response to ACTH stimulation (Fig. 4). This is an important condition to keep in mind when looking into therapeutic choices [43]. To better understand how the adrenal gland acts, a study on the co-secretion of gonadotropins with androgen (androstenedione) and cortisol with androgens (androstenedione) was conducted on two groups of PCOS patients: one hyperandrogenic from ovarian overproduction and the other hyperandrogenic from stress-induced hyperproduction.

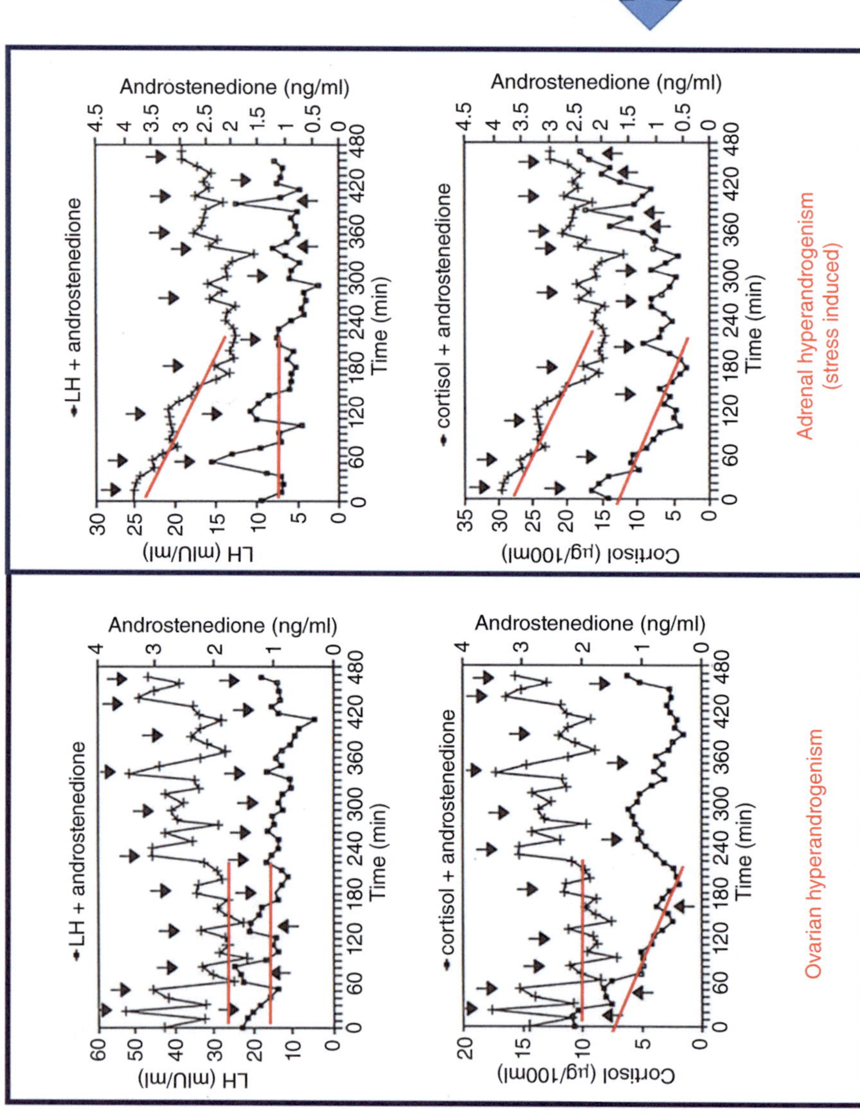

Fig. 4 Hyperandrogenism might be related also to a temporary adrenal hyperfunction. When stress is present, cortisol and androstenedione profiles show a parallel trend as in the lower panel on the right. In case stress is not so intense, LH drives androstenedione secretion from the ovary, and both hormones show a parallel trend (upper panel on the left). (Modified from ref. 44)

In the first group, the LH and androstenedione plasma profiles were found to be co-secreted, showing a parallel trend. Since LH drives the ovary, androstenedione peaks are co-secreted with those of LH, thus indicating that this androgen is predominantly with an ovarian origin (Fig. 4).

The other group of patients showed the opposite situation: while the LH pulsatile profile did not show variability, the androstenedione profile decreased its plasma levels within 2 h from the beginning of the test, and, in addition, the profiles of cortisol and androstenedione showed a parallel trend, both starting high at the beginning of the test and then lowering in a parallel manner, with cortisol and androstenedione pulses being co-secreted (Fig. 4). This indicates that, although a part of androstenedione had an ovarian origin, in these patients, a greater part comes from the hyperactivated adrenal gland [44].

It is also important to consider that adrenal hyperandrogenism should be suspected when elevated DHEAS and 17-OHP basal hormone levels are found together with androstenedione; due to an enzymatic defect of the adrenal gland, hyperandrogenism arises from the deficiency of one of these enzymes: 21-hydroxylase, 11β-hydroxylase, or 3β/-hydroxysteroid-dehydrogenase.

With these enzyme defects, the adrenal gland tries to arrive at the synthesis of cortisol through other pathways, but this leads to the excess of the intermediate products upstream of cortisol, leading to a greater release of DHEAS, 17-OHP, and androstenedione. Despite the fact that PCOS is 40–50 times more frequent than non-classic congenital adrenal hyperplasia (NC-CAH) in fertile women than in women with hyperandrogenism, it is essential to check for NC-CAH in all patients with apparent PCOS [45, 46]. Levels of 17-OHP, DHEAS, androstenedione, and cortisol plasma have to be checked. In the case that cortisol is normal, but 17-OHP and androstenedione are too high, an issue at the adrenal gland is suspected [23].

Plasma levels of 17-OHP above 200 ng/dL (6 nmol/L) strongly indicate the presence of NC-CAH, whereas plasma concentrations below 200 ng/dL (6 nmol/L) do not sustain the presence of NC-CAH. To prove the suspicion, an ACTH stimulation test has to be performed. A 17-OHP response equal or higher than 1500 ng/dL (43 nmol/L) under ACTH stimulation confirms the suspicion of NC-CAH [47, 48].

With 17-OHP plasma levels being increased during the preovulatory or luteal phase of the menstrual cycle, plasma evaluation has to be performed no later than 8–10 days after the beginning of the menstrual bleeding or any time if the patient is amenorrheic.

The final result, independently from the origin of hyperandrogenism, is that an altered GnRH-gonadotropin secretion occurs with no chance for follicles to develop and/or mature and oligo-/amenorrhea takes place.

6 Prolactin

Prolactin (PRL) is a protein hormone that stimulates milk production in female mammals [49]. PRL release is in a pulsatile manner and modulates metabolism, the immune system, and pancreatic development.

PRL also acts as a neuropeptide when it crosses the blood-brain barrier: it gets though a PRLRs-independent mechanism and modulates the hypothalamus, central functions, behavior, arousal, and sexuality [50, 51].

PRL is under the control of the tuberoinfundibular dopaminergic system (TIDA) that directly controls PRL release from the gonadotropes inhibiting PRL secretion [52]. Though mostly released by the anterior pituitary, PRL has also extra-pituitary origins such as from the brain, prostate, immune cells, skin, adipose tissue, and human decidua [49]. PRL secretion also depends from the direct stimulation of TRH that classically controls TSH secretion and thyroid function [53]. Despite being secreted by different cells, prolactin and TSH are related, since they are both stimulated by thyrotropin-releasing hormone (TRH). In the presence of any functional defect that induces hypothyroidism, TSH is higher due to an increase in the release of TRH at the hypothalamic level, and, consequently, PRL becomes higher. PRL reaches the target cells through the circulatory system and acts on specific receptors, located on the cell membrane [54].

With no endocrine target organ to provide feedback control, the biological evolution of PRL made it regulate its own secretion within the hypothalamus, modulating the hypothalamic releasing and inhibiting factors that control their secretions. PRL suppresses its own secretion acting on tuberoinfundibular (TIDA) neurons located in the arcuate nucleus that stimulate the synthesis and release of dopamine into the portal vessels at the median eminence [55]. Dopamine acts on D2 receptors to inhibit PRL synthesis and release. In addition to TRH, other PRL-releasing factors are serotonin (5-HT), vasoactive intestinal peptide (VIP), and arginine vasopressin (AVP) [56].

PRL is a putative disruptor of the normal neuroendocrine control of the ovarian cycle. Therefore, it is one of the many hormones involved in the control of follicle maturation, in the evolution of the luteal phase, in the interference of FSH-induced aromatization, and in the modulation of GnRH secretion.

Together with DA, PRL exerts negative feedback on its secretion and GnRH production, thus explaining how hyperprolactinemia interferes with human reproduction [49]. An excess of PRL up to the extent of hyperprolactinemia can interfere with reproduction. Hyperprolactinemia decreases GnRH and, subsequently, LH secretion, decreasing pulse frequency and amplitude, thus affecting gonadal steroid production and inducing menstrual irregularities.

The effects of PRL on fertility have been studied in animal models that confirmed that reproduction needs PRL signaling. Both short and long isoforms of PRLRs are expressed by the granulosa, interstitial, and luteal cells at the ovarian level, as well as in the endometrium, myometrium, and decidua in the uterus.

Kisspeptin-secreting neurons are essential for pubertal maturation in humans and are the main inductors of GnRH secretion. Kisspeptin is probably involved as a potential mediator of prolactin's actions on fertility [57]. Kisspeptin and prolactin are able to modulate each other, but in different ways according to the species. In fact, kisspeptin induces PRL prolactin release in rats when estradiol levels are high, while in women, the concomitant pulsatile release of PRL with kisspeptin-induced LH occurs when they are hypogonadal [53, 58].

In response to stress, PRL acts negatively on the hypothalamic-pituitary axis, modulating GnRH release as well as the adrenal activity through the modulation of corticotropin-releasing hormone (CRH)-ACTH secretions [50].

PRL is linked to emotional responsiveness, acting on the modulation of anxiety and depressive disorders in female mice. Acute stressor events suppress the activation of kisspeptin neurons, and LH pulsatile release is reduced. When the same stress is chronically administered during the day, mice showed higher corticosterone levels and the lengthening of the estrous cycles. Such chronic stressor situations can induce hyperprolactinemia, thus participating to impaired fertility in women [59, 60].

PRL promotes also leptin resistance and increased appetite, hyperphagia, and insulin resistance: under pathological hyperprolactinemia, obesity, abnormal glucose tolerance, and hyperinsulinemia due to insulin resistance have been observed.

Weight gain (up to obesity) and insulin resistance occur frequently when PRL plasma levels are 70–100 ng/mL or higher: this tends to occur during hyperprolactinemia due to pituitary adenomas, hypothyroidism, or under specific medications (i.e., antidepressants, prokinetics, antipsychotics).

Circulating levels of PRL in women are usually around 10–15 ng/mL: when these levels are above 25 ng/mL, they are conventionally defined as hyperprolactinemia [49]. Recently, it has been reported that patients suffering from polycystic ovary syndrome (PCOS) have higher PRL levels (18–20 ng/mL), despite not having hyperprolactinemia. In the case of stress (fear, psychological stress, etc.), PRL plasma levels increase rapidly (up to 90–100 ng/mL) [61].

Lifestyle, body mass index (BMI), excessive physical activity, and stressful situations have to be monitored. If PRL plasma levels are above 50 ng/mL, a pituitary magnetic resonance imaging (MRI), preferably enhanced with gadolinium, should be performed in order to disclose the presence of a pituitary adenoma or any other sellar/parasellar mass, which might be causing stalk compression [61, 62].

In general, hyperprolactinemia around or above 50 up to 100 ng/mL is a possible indicator of a secreting adenoma; untreated hypothyroidism can rarely also mimic an adenoma: this requires TSH to be checked [49] (Fig. 5). In the case of dysfunctional hyperprolactinemia, the treatment is quite simple: cabergoline decreases prolactin levels slowly, decreases androgens in circulation, and increases gonadotropins. As a dopamine agonist, cabergoline is better than bromocriptine in controlling PRL levels in hyperprolactinemic men and women with sexual dysfunctions [49].

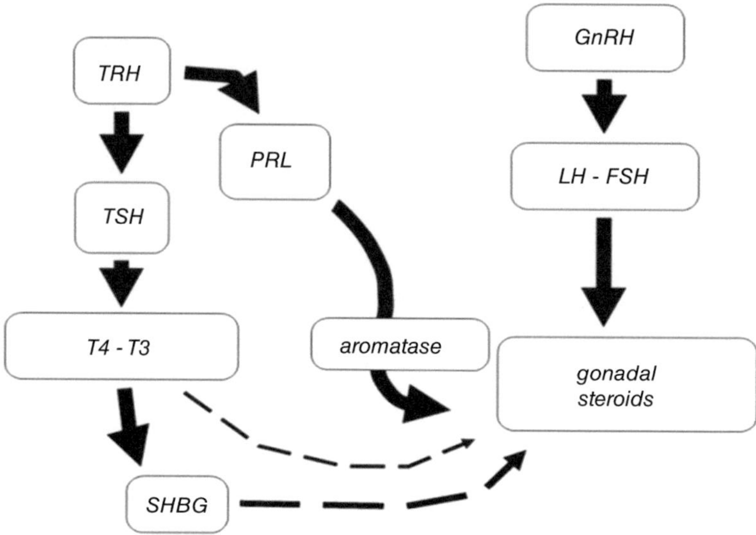

Fig. 5 The interconnection between PRL and thyroid axes. TRH is able to induce both PRL and TSH secretion

7 Thyroid

The thyroidal axis is one of the primary endocrine axes for mammals. Thyroid diseases are quite frequent, more common in women than men, and they may interfere with the reproductive system [63].

Hyperthyroidism can impair menstrual bleeding, inducing hypomenorrhea and polymenorrhea, while hypothyroidism induces oligomenorrhea and sometimes these menstrual irregularities occur prior to the identification of thyroid disease [64]. Thyroid hormones can impair reproduction, increasing liver production of sex hormone-binding globulin (SHBG) and of ovarian testosterone and androstenedione secretion, reducing the clearance of all gonadal steroids, and accelerating the conversion of androgens to estrone.

Receptors for thyroid hormones are at the level of oocytes, where these hormones act synergically with FSH to induce the production of sexual hormones [65]. Thyroid dysfunctions result in the high frequency of abnormal menstrual bleeding due to ovulatory impairments. In fact, triiodothyronine (T3) acts on folliculogenesis, modulating the P13K/Akt pathway [66]. Due to this, hypothyroidism is associated with a reduced fertility rate despite the recognition of the endometrial expression of deiodinase type 3 and placental increases in T3 [67, 68].

Estrogens also increase the concentrations of thyroxine binding globulin (TBG) [69]. TBG concentrations increase greatly with the menopausal transition during menopause and later with the aging process, as well as for the hypoestrogenic condition [70]. Main causes of hypothyroidism are iodine deficiency and autoimmune thyroiditis; it can also occur due to iodine therapy for thyroid cancer, thyroidectomy, and rare diseases (such as scleroderma and amyloidosis) [71, 72].

Other reasons are lithium treatment or iodine-containing drugs. The symptoms of hypothyroidism are lethargy, pretibial myxedema, hypothermia, and the tendency to gain weight due to the accumulation of sugar derivatives that are deposited in the extracellular matrix adsorbing water.

Chronic condition of hypothyroidism with high antibodies correlates with a greater risk of early ovarian failure in 15% of cases, together with higher incidence of anti-thyroid and anti-ovarian antibodies [1].

Oligomenorrhea is the classic menstrual abnormality induced by hypothyroidism that may be diagnosed for the highest TSH plasma levels. This is very frequent in the case of recurrent abortion. At the basis of the infertility state induced by hypothyroidism are the impaired peripheral estrogen metabolism, the presence of hyperprolactinemia, and abnormal GnRH secretion that affect gonadotropin secretions [73]. Due to the slowing of the metabolic clearance of gonadal steroids, hypothyroidism increases androstenedione and estrone plasma levels and permits the increase in peripheral aromatization [55, 56]. Moreover, with SHBG being decreased, both total testosterone and E2, unbound fractions are increased. Impairments of steroid metabolism disappear when a euthyroid state is restored with an appropriate treatment [74].

Thyroid autoimmunity is the most frequent autoimmune disease (5–20%) in fertile women and is the cause of hypothyroid function; it is characterized by the presence of anti-thyroid antibodies. One kind of antibodies (anti-TSH) has an allosteric conformation similar to TSH and for this reason can bind to the receptor by inducing high fT3 and fT4; for the diagnosis, it is important to assay these antibodies in the plasma [23].

Thyroid autoimmunity is more common in females than in males and is related to the action of both estrogens and androgens on the immune system. Early menarche or a late menopause is considered a risk factor for the development of an autoimmune thyroiditis, probably due to the long exposure to estrogen during the reproductive life [75, 76]. Symptoms can simulate the onset of early menopause since antibodies against the ovary might produce hot flashes, amenorrhea, moodiness, and insomnia.

Hyperthyroidism classically shows undetectable levels of serum TSH and elevated FT3 and FT4 concentrations. In subclinical hyperthyroidism, the serum TSH level is low or very low, but FT3 and FT4 concentrations are normal.

The most frequent cause of hyperthyroidism is Graves' disease. On the contrary, Plummer toxic adenoma and toxic multinodular goiter are highly frequent where iodine intake is low [77]. Graves' disease is triggered by the high synthesis of an immunoglobulin that binds the TSH receptor. The toxic adenomas can induce thyrotoxicosis due to the growth of benign monoclonal thyroid cells able to hyperproduce thyroid hormones. Usually, only a single functioning nodule develops, but in some cases more than one nodule can grow (toxic multinodular goiter), and this is more frequent after the age of 60 [74]. Sometimes, thyrotoxicosis starts after a postpartum thyroiditis or subacute thyroiditis or due to unintentional excessive replacement therapy in hypothyroid subjects or to intentional TSH suppressive therapy for benign or malignant thyroid disease. The hypersecretion of TSH for a trophoblastic tumor or metastatic thyroid carcinoma is very rare. Amenorrhea is a classic and precocious symptom associated with hyperthyroidism [75]. Together with thyrotoxicosis there is the increase in serum levels of SHBG and also frequently of estrogen during all phases of the menstrual cycle (compared with normal women) [76].

This is because the metabolic clearance rate of estradiol is reduced in hyperthyroidism, and this is related to the increased binding of E2 to SHBG [77].

Androgen metabolism also changes, since plasma levels of testosterone and androstenedione are increased together with higher production rates. The increased estrogenic tone is also sustained by the higher conversion rate of androstenedione to estrone and of testosterone to E2, thus participating in the maintenance of the impaired gonadotropin secretion all along the menstrual cycle [78, 79]. LH plasma levels are increased; on the contrary, the pulsatile secretion does not differ. Once treatment is started with antithyroid drugs, LH goes back to normal levels [80].

It is relevant to point out that thyroid dysregulation often induces a PCO-like panel. Though it cannot be excluded a possible link due to common factors, the feature of the impaired androgenic milieu that hyperthyroidism may show is at the basis of such morphology at the ultrasound scan.

Hashimoto's thyroiditis (HT) triggers metabolic impairments due to the thyroid dysfunction; similarly, insulin resistance may occur and, if combined with a PCOS, may worsen to cardiovascular risks. The coexistence of HT and PCOS may exaggerate metabolic dysfunctions that usually might be spread by higher values of body weight, glucose level, insulin, HOMA-IR index, and lipid profile [81].

If a thyroid dysfunction is suspected, fT3, fT4, and TSH should be controlled together with the antibodies' plasma levels; in the case that TSH is very low, anti-TSH antibodies must be assayed, and an ultrasound scan of the thyroid gland has to be performed. If a defect of fT3 is found, we have to exclude hypothyroidism. This is the case of stress-induced amenorrhea when the "low T3 syndrome" is triggered and the activity of the thyroid gland is decreased by reducing the T4 toT3 conversion, with normal TSH plasma levels. This happens because a distinct deiodinase, activated in these cases, leads to the synthesis of a biologically inactive T3, called reverse T3 (rT3). In these patients levothyroxine should not be administered, since the low fT3 level is a defensive event to prevent excess energy consumption. Additionally, the metabolic profile and the hormonal basal levels of the reproductive axis should be analyzed in order to find the primary cause of the hormonal disease [23].

In conclusion normal reproductive function is affected by all the clinical pathophysiological situations described. Ovarian function is dependent on the equilibrium among the many endocrine and neuroendocrine factors so as to modulate the hypothalamic centers where the reproductive function is triggered controlling follicle recruitment and maturation.

References

1. Yen SSC, Jaffe RB. Reproductive endocrinology: physiology, pathophysiology, and clinical management. Philadelphia, PA: Elsevier; 2017.
2. Podfigurna A, Maciejewska-Jeske M, Meczekalski B, Genazzani AD. Kisspeptin and LH pulsatility in patients with functional hypothalamic amenorrhea. Endocrine. 2020;70:635–43.
3. Meczekalski B, Katulski K, Czyzyk A, Podfigurna-Stopa A, MacIejewska-Jeske M. Functional hypothalamic amenorrhea and its influence on women's health. J Endocrinol Investig. 2014;37(11):1049.
4. Genazzani AD, Podfigurna A, Szeliga A, Meczekalski B. Kisspeptin in female reproduction: from physiology to pathophysiology. Gynecol Reprod Endocrinol Metab. 2021;2(3):148–55.
5. Gordon CM, Ackerman KE, Berga SL, Kaplan JR, Mastorakos G, Misra M, Murad MH, Santoro NF, Warren MO. Functional hypothalamic amenorrhea: an Endocrine Society clinical practice guideline. J Clin Endocrinol Metab. 2017;102(5):1413–39.
6. Bergadà C, Moguilevsky JA, editors. Ares-Serono Symposia Publication: Rome, Italy; 1995.
7. Genazzani AD. Neuroendocrine aspects of amenorrhea related to stress. Pediatr Endocrinol Rev. 2005;2:661–8.
8. Genazzani AD, Despini G, Prati A, Manzo A, Petrillo T, Tomatis V, Giannini A, Simoncini T. Administration of very low doses of estradiol modulates the LH response to a GnRH bolus and the LH and cortisol responses to naloxone infusion in patients with functional hypothalamic amenorrhea (FHA): a pilot study. Endocrine. 2020;1(1):35–45.
9. Genazzani AD, Santagni S, Chierchia E, Rattighieri E, Campedelli A, Prati A, Ricchieri F, Simoncini T. Estimation of instantaneous secretory rates and intrinsic characteristics of luteinizing hormone secretion in women with Kallmann syndrome before and after estriol administration. Reprod Biol. 2011;11(3):284–93.
10. Genazzani AD, Meczekalski B, Podfigurna-Stopa A, Santagni S, Rattighieri E, Ricchieri F, Chierchia E, Simoncini T. Estriol administration modulates luteinizing hormone secretion in women with functional hypothalamic amenorrhea. Fertil Steril. 2012;97(2):483–8.
11. Genazzani AD, Chierchia E, Santagni S, Rattighieri E, Farinetti A, Lanzoni C. Hypothalamic amenorrhea: from diagnosis to therapeutical approach. Ann Endocrinol (Paris). 2010;71(3):163–9.
12. Facchinetti F, Fava M, Fioroni L, Genazzani AD, Genazzani AR. Stressful life events and affective disorders inhibit pulsatile LH secretion in hypothalamic amenorrhea. Psychoneuroendocrinology. 1993;18(5–6):397–404.
13. Rivier C, Rivier J, Vale W. Stress-induced inhibition of reproductive functions: role of endogenous corticotropin-releasing factor. Science. 1986;231(4738):607–9.
14. Genazzani AD, Petraglia F, Gastaldi M, Volpogni C, D'Ambrogio G, Facchinetti F, Genazzani AR. FSH secretory pattern and degree of concordance with LH in amenorrheic, fertile, and postmenopausal women. Am J Phys. 1993;264:E776–81.
15. Genazzani AD, Petraglia F, Fabbri G, Monzani A, Montanini V, Genazzani AR. Evidence of luteinizing hormone secretion in hypothalamic amenorrhea associated with weight loss. Fertil Steril. 1990;54(2):222–6.
16. Genazzani AD, Petraglia F, Benatti R, Montanini V, Algeri I, Annible V, Genazzani AR. Luteinizing hormone (LH) secretory burst duration is independent from LH, prolactin, or gonadal steroid plasma levels in amenorrheic women. J Clin Endocrinol Metab. 1991;72(6):1220–5.
17. Genazzani AD, Petraglia F, Volpogni C, Gastaldi M, Pianazzi F, Montanini V, Genazzani AR. Modulatory role of estrogens and progestins on growth hormone episodic release in women with hypothalamic amenorrhea. Fertil Steril. 1993;60(3):465–70.
18. Genazzani AD, Petraglia F, Algeri I, Gastaldi M, Calvani M, Bogticelli G, Genazzani AR. Acetyl-L-carnitine as possible drug in the treatment of hypothalamic amenorrhea. Acta Obstet Gynecol Scand. 1991;70(6):487–92.

19. Kalogeras KT, Calogero AE, Kuribayiashi T, Khan I, Gallucci WT, Kling MA, Chrousos GP, Gold PW. In vitro and in vivo effects of triazolobenzodiazepine alprazolam and hypothalamic-pituitary-adrenal function: pharmacological and clinical implications. J Clin Endocrinol Metab. 1990;70(5):1462–71.
20. Batrinos ML, Panitsa-Faflia C, Courcoutsakis N, Chatzipavlou V. Incidence, type, and etiology of menstrual disorders in the age group 12–19 years. Adolesc Pediatr Gynecol. 1990;3(3):149–53.
21. Frisch RE, McArthur JW. Menstrual cycles: fatness as a determinant of minimum weight for height necessary for their maintenance or onset. Science. 1974;185(4155):949–51.
22. Genazzani AR, Petraglia F, Gamba O, Sgarbi L, Greco MM, Genazzani AD. Neuroendocrinology of the menstrual cycle. Gynecol Endosc Surg. 1994:48–54.
23. Genazzani AD, Santagni S, Rattighieri E, Chierchia E, Despini G, Prati A, Ricchieri F. PCOS and insulin resistance (IR): from lifestyle to insulin sensitizers. Int Soc Gynecol Endocrinol Ser. 2015:11–23.
24. Genazzani AD, Despini G, Bonacini R, Prati A. Functional hypothalamic amenorrhea as stress induced defensive system. Int Soc Gynecol Endocrinol Ser. 2017:111–8.
25. Genazzani AD, Prati A, Simoncini T, Napolitano A. Modulatory role of D-chiro-inositol and alpha lipoic acid combination on hormonal and metabolic parameters of overweight/obese PCOS patients. Eur Gynecol Obs. 2019;1:29–33.
26. Skorupskaite K, George JT, Anderson RA. The kisspeptin-GnRH pathway in human reproductive health and disease. Hum Reprod Update. 2014;20(4):485–500.
27. Hall JE. The female reproductive system, infertility and contraception. In: Harrison's endocrinology. New York: McGraw-Hill Education; 2011. p. 178–93.
28. Fourman LT, Fazeli PK. Neuroendocrine causes of amenorrhea—an update. J Clin Endocrinol Metab. 2015;100(3):812–24.
29. Frisch RE. Body fat, puberty and fertility. Biol Rev. 1984;59(2):161–88.
30. Reid RL, Van Vugt DA. Weight-related changes in reproductive function. Fertil Steril. 1987;48(6):905–13.
31. Joseph D, Whirledge S. Stress and the HPA axis: balancing homeostasis and fertility. Int J Mol Sci. 2017;18(10):2224.
32. Astapova O, Minor BMN, Hammes SR. Physiological and pathological androgen actions in the ovary. Endocrinology. 2019;160(5):1166–74.
33. Sen A, Hammes SR. Granulosa cell-specific androgen receptors are critical regulators of ovarian development and function. Mol Endocrinol. 2010;24(7):1393–403.
34. Whirledge S, Cidlowski JA. Glucocorticoids and reproduction: traffic control on the road to reproduction. Trends Endocrinol Metab. 2017;28(6):399–415.
35. Magiakou MA, Mastorakos G, Webster E, Chrousos GP. The hypothalamic-pituitary-adrenal axis and the female reproductive system. Ann N Y Acad Sci. 1997;816(1):42–56.
36. Barbarino A, De Marinis L, Tofani A, Della Casa S, D'Amico C, Mancini A, Corsello SM, Sciuto R, Barini A. Corticotropin-releasing hormone inhibition of gonadotropin release and the effect of opioid blockade. J Clin Endocrinol Metab. 1989;68(3):523–8.
37. Ortega MT, McGrath JA, Carlson L, Poccia VF, Gary Larson CD, Sun BZ, Zhao S, Beery B, Vesper HW, Duke L, Botelho JC, Filie AC, Shaw ND. Longitudinal investigation of pubertal milestones and hormones as a function of body fat in girls. J Clin Endocrinol Metab. 2021;106(6):1668–83.
38. Genazzani AD. Inositol as putative integrative treatment for PCOS. Reprod Biomed Online. 2016;33(6):770–80.
39. Fauser BCJM, Tarlatzis BC, Rebar RW, Legro RS, Balen AH, Lobo R, et al. Consensus on women's health aspects of polycystic ovary syndrome (PCOS): the Amsterdam ESHRE/ASRM-Sponsored 3rd PCOS Consensus Workshop Group. Fertil Steril. 2012;97(1):28.
40. Genazzani AD, Prati A, Chierchia E, Santagni S. Gli stati iperandrogenici. Boll Ginecol Endocrinol. 2014;8:35–44.

41. Genazzani AD. Expert's opinion: integrative treatment with inositols and lipoic acid for insulin resistance of PCOS. Gynecol Reprod Endocrinol Metab. 2020:146–57.
42. Lizneva D, Gavrilova-Jordan L, Walker W, Azziz R. Androgen excess: investigations and management. Best Pract Res Clin Obstet Gynaecol. 2016;37:98–118.
43. Farah-Eways L, Reyna R, Knochenhauer ES, Bartolucci AA, Azziz R. Glucose action and adrenocortical biosynthesis in women with polycystic ovary syndrome. Fertil Steril. 2004;81(1):120–5.
44. Genazzani AD, Petraglia F, Pianazzi F, Volpogni C, Genazzani AR. The concomitant release of androstenedione with cortisol and luteinizing hormone pulsatile releases distinguishes adrenal from ovarian hyperandrogenism. Gynecol Endocrinol. 1993;7(1):33–41.
45. Moran C, Azziz R. 21-Hydroxylase-deficient nonclassic adrenal hyperplasia: the great pretender. Semin Reprod Med. 2003;21(3):295–300.
46. Ding T, Hardiman PJ, Petersen I, Wang FF, Qu F, Baio G. The prevalence of polycystic ovary syndrome in reproductive-aged women of different ethnicity: a systematic review and meta-analysis. Oncotarget. 2017;8(56):96351–8.
47. Speiser PW, Azziz R, Baskin LS, Ghizzoni L, Hensle TW, Merke DP, Meyer Bahlburg HFL, Miller WL, Montori VM, Oberfield SE, Ritzen M, White PC, Perrin C, et al. Congenital adrenal hyperplasia due to steroid 21-hydroxylase deficiency: an Endocrine Society clinical practice guideline. J Clin Endocrinol Metab. 2010;95(9):4133–60.
48. Azziz R, Dewailly D, Owerbach D. Clinical review 56: nonclassic adrenal hyperplasia: current concepts. J Clin Endocrinol Metab. 1994;78(4):810–5.
49. Nappi RE, Di Ciaccio S, Genazzani AD. Prolactin as a neuroendocrine clue in sexual function of women across the reproductive life cycle: an expert point of view. Gynecol Endocrinol. 2021;37(6):490–6.
50. Suchecki D, Elias CF, Makara GB, Torner L. Actions of prolactin in the brain: from physiological adaptations to stress and neurogenesis to psychopathology. Front Endocrinol (Lausanne). 2016;7:25.
51. Brown RSE, Wyatt AK, Herbison RE, Knowles PJ, Ladyman SR, Binart N, Banks WA, Grattan DR. Prolactin transport into mouse brain is independent of prolactin receptor. FASEB J. 2016;30(2):1002–10.
52. Timmerman W, Deinum ME, Poelman RT, Westerink BH, Schuiling GA. Characterisation of the DA-ergic system in the mediobasal hypothalamus: a new approach to simultaneously monitor the release of DA from the TIDA neurons and the PRL secretion from the adenohypophysis in awake rats. Brain Res. 1994;657(1/2):275–80.
53. Cetel NS, Yen SSC. Concomitant pulsatile release of prolactin and luteinizing hormone in hypogonadal women. J Clin Endocrinol Metab. 1983;56(6):1313–5.
54. Bole-Feysot C, Goffin V, Edery M, Binart N, Kelly PA. Prolactin (PRL) and its receptor: actions, signal transduction pathways and phenotypes observed in PRL receptor knockout mice. Endocr Rev. 1998;19(3):225–68.
55. Leong DA, Frawley LS, Neill JD. Neuroendocrine control of prolactin secretion. Annu Rev Physiol. 1983;45:109–27.
56. Melmed S, Polonsky KS, Larsen PR, Kronenberg HM. Williams textbook of endocrinology. 13th ed. Amsterdam: Elsevier; 2015.
57. de Roux N, Genin E, Carel J-C, Matsuda F, Chaussain J-L, Milgrom E. Hypogonadotropic hypogonadism due to loss of function of the KiSS1-derived peptide receptor GPR54. Proc Natl Acad Sci U S A. 2003;100:10972.
58. Ribeiro AB, Leite CM, Kalil B, Franci CR, Anselmo-Franci JA, Szawka RE. Kisspeptin regulates tuberoinfundibular dopaminergic neurones and prolactin secretion in an oestradiol-dependent manner in male and female rats. J Neuroendocrinol. 2015;27(2):88–99.
59. Yang JA, Song CI, Hughes JK, Kreisman MJ, Parra RA, Haisenleder DJ, Kauffman AS, Breen KM. Acute psychosocial stress inhibits LH pulsatility and Kiss1 neuronal activation in female mice. Endocrinology. 2017;158(11):3716–23.

60. Levine S, Muneyyirci-Delale O. Stress-induced hyperprolactinemia: pathophysiology and clinical approach. Obstet Gynecol Int. 2018;2018:1.
61. Melmed S, Casanueva FF, Hoffman AR, Kleinberg DL, Montori VM, Schlechte JA, Wass JAH. Diagnosis and treatment of hyperprolactinemia: an Endocrine Society clinical practice guideline. J Clin Endocrinol Metab. 2011;96(2):273–88.
62. Kalsi AK, Halder A, Jain M, Chaturvedi PK, Sharma JB. Prevalence and reproductive manifestations of macroprolactinemia. Endocrine. 2019;63(2):332–40.
63. Poppe K, Velkeniers B, Glinoer D. Thyroid disease and female reproduction. Clin Endocrinol. 2007;66(3):309–21.
64. Krassas GE, Poppe K, Glinoer D. Thyroid function and human reproductive health. Endocr Rev. 2010;31(5):702–55.
65. Cecconi S, Rucci N, Scaldaferri ML, Masciulli MP, Rossi G, Moretti C, D'Armiento M, Ulisse S. Thyroid hormone effects on mouse oocyte maturation and granulosa cell aromatase activity. Endocrinology. 1999;140(9):1783–8.
66. Zhang C, Guo L, Zhu B, Feng Y, Yu S, An N, Wang X. Effects of 3, 5, 3′-triiodothyronine (t3) and follicle stimulating hormone on apoptosis and proliferation of rat ovarian granulosa cells. Chin J Physiol. 2013;56(5):298–305.
67. Korevaar TIM, Medici M, Visser TJ, Peeters RP. Thyroid disease in pregnancy: new insights in diagnosis and clinical management. Nat Rev Endocrinol. 2017;13(10):610–22.
68. Huang SA, Dorfman DM, Genest DR, Salvatore D, Larsen PR. Type 3 iodothyronine deiodinase is highly expressed in the human uteroplacental unit and in fetal epithelium. J Clin Endocrinol Metab. 2003;88(3):1384–8.
69. Ain KB, Mori Y, Refetoff S. Reduced clearance rate of thyroxine-binding globulin (TBG) with increased sialylation: a mechanism for estrogen-induced elevation of serum TBG concentration. J Clin Endocrinol Metab. 1987;65(4):689–96.
70. Meldrum D, Defazio J, Erlik Y, Lu J, Wolfsen AF, Carlson H, Hershman J, Judd H. Pituitary hormones during the menopausal hot flash. Obstet Gynecol. 1984;64(6):752–6.
71. Zimmermann MB, Andersson M. Assessment of iodine nutrition in populations: past, present, and future. Nutr Rev. 2012;70(10):553–70.
72. Vanderpump MPJ, Tunbridge WMG, French JM, Appleton D, Bates D, Clark F. The incidence of thyroid disorders in the community: a twenty-year follow-up of the Whickham Survey. Clin Endocrinol. 1995;43(1):55–68.
73. Krassas GE. Thyroid disease and female reproduction. Fertil Steril. 2000;74(6):1063–70.
74. Gordon GG, Southren AL. Thyroid - hormone effects on steroid—hormone metabolism. Bull N Y Acad Med. 1977;53(3):241–59.
75. Phillips DIW, Lazarus JH, Butland BK. The influence of pregnancy and reproductive span on the occurrence of autoimmune thyroiditis. Clin Endocrinol. 1990;32(3):301–6.
76. Sawin CT, Castelli WP, Hershman JM, McNamara P, Bacharach P. The aging thyroid: thyroid deficiency in the Framingham study. Arch Intern Med. 1985;145(8):1386–8.
77. Carlé A, Pedersen IB, Knudsen N, Perrild H, Oversen L, Rasmussen LB, Laurberg P. Epidemiology of subtypes of hyperthyroidism in Denmark: a population-based study. Eur J Endocrinol. 2011;164(5):801–9.
78. The male and female reproductive system in thyrotoxicosis—Werner & Ingbar's the thyroid: a fundamental & clinical text, 9th ed. https://doctorlib.info/medical/thyroid/50.html. Accessed 15 Nov 2022.
79. Akande EO, Hockaday TDR. Plasma luteinizing hormone levels in women with thyrotoxicosis. J Endocrinol. 1972;53(1):173–4.
80. Akande EO. The effect of oestrogen on plasma levels of luteinizing hormone in euthyroid and thyrotoxic postmenopausal women. Int J Obstet Gynaecol. 1974;81(10):795–803.
81. Ganie MA, Marwaha RK, Aggarwal R, Singh S. High prevalence of polycystic ovary syndrome characteristics in girls with euthyroid chronic lymphocytic thyroiditis: a case-control study. Eur J Endocrinol. 2010;162(6):1117–22.

Luteal Phase Defects

Johannes Ott, Iris Holzer, and Christian Goebl

1 Introduction

The female reproductive processes are characterized by an inconstant activity of the hypothalamus-pituitary-gonadal axis. Within these physiologic processes, accurate timing is necessary to achieve the ultimate goal, namely, live birth [1]. This chapter will be about the luteal phase of the menstrual cycle, which is traditionally called the "second half" of the cycle. After some relevant physiologic considerations, the focus will be on luteal phase defects in general, in special situations and in the course of artificial reproduction.

2 Specific Physiologic Considerations

2.1 The Model of "Follicular Waves"

In the traditional model, during the late luteal phase, a single cohort, consisting of 3–11 follicles, is recruited to grow in each ovary. From this cohort, a single dominant follicle seems to get selected, which then continues to develop during the follicular phase and eventually ovulates, while the other follicles regress. After ovulation, during the early and mid-luteal phase, it was believed that follicular quiescence would occur, mainly due to the inhibitory effects of luteal progesterone

J. Ott (✉) · I. Holzer · C. Goebl
Clinical Division of Gynecologic Endocrinology and Reproductive Medicine, Medical University of Vienna, Vienna, Austria
e-mail: johannes.ott@meduniwien.ac.at; iris.holzer@meduniwien.ac.at; christian.goebl@meduniwien.ac.at

A. R. Genazzani et al. (eds.), *Menstrual Bleeding and Pain Disorders from Adolescence to Menopause*, ISGE Series,
https://doi.org/10.1007/978-3-031-55300-4_7

production [2–5]. However, it has become clear that in fact more than only one, namely, two to three "waves" of follicles, grow per cycle, which is the case in about two and three thirds of women, respectively [5, 6]. A "wave" is defined as the synchronous growth of a group, i.e., a cohort of antral follicles [5]. The first of two or the first two of three waves grow in the luteal phase. Usually only the last wave, which corresponds to the single cohort of the traditional model, grows during the follicular phase and reaches ovulation [6]. These waves can be classified into major and minor waves, according to whether a dominant follicle would grow, and into ovulatory and non-ovulatory waves. Ovulatory waves only occur in major waves, i.e., waves with a dominant follicle [5, 6] (Fig. 1).

According to this model, there are dominant follicles in both the follicular and the luteal phase (FDPF, follicular phase dominant follicle; LPDF, luteal phase dominant follicle). Concerning the endocrine processes in the luteal phase, it has been demonstrated in women of mid-reproductive age that LPDFs were associated with higher estradiol levels, whereas they did not have an influence on progesterone levels. Thus, it is believed that the source of progesterone is only the corpus luteum, whereas estradiol is derived from the corpus luteum and the LPDF. Moreover, notwithstanding some estradiol production by the corpus luteum, the levels are more consistent with the notion of a follicular origin [7]. This also explains the association between the rise in follicular stimulating hormone (FSH) and the rise in

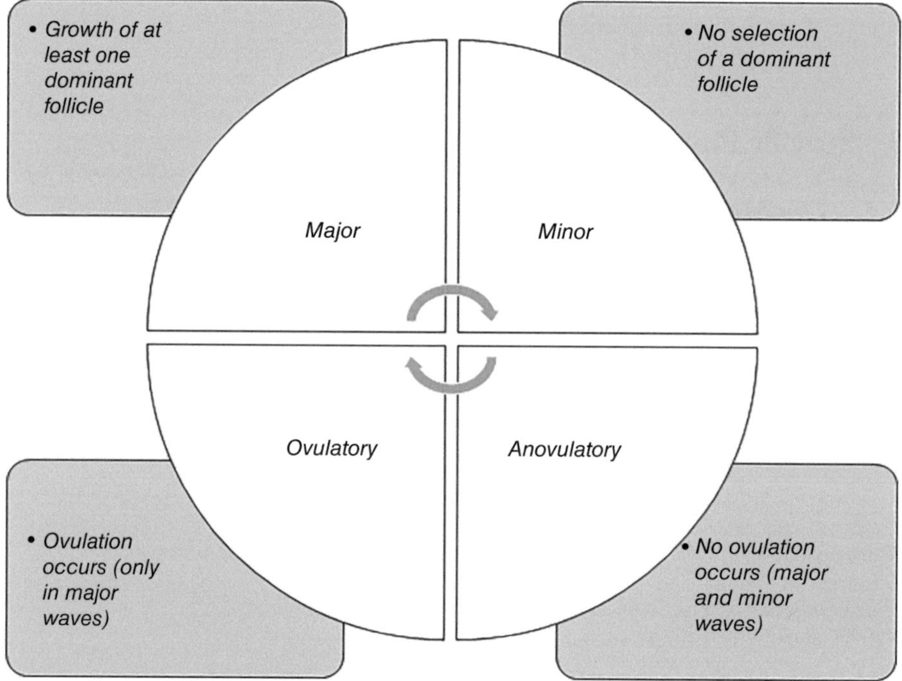

Fig. 1 Classification of follicular waves

estradiol in the luteal phase, since the emergence of both major and minor follicular waves is always preceded by an increase in FSH [5, 6]. Last not least, LPDFs are associated with higher inhibin B levels which source seems to be that LPDF as well as the new emerging cohort [7].

2.2 The Source of Progesterone Production

It has been demonstrated that, due to a rise in GnRH, LH is rising in the luteal phase, which is necessary for an increase in progesterone secretion [8]. However, there are two sources of progesterone in the corpus luteum: first, the small luteal cells, which originate from the granulosa cells, contribute to progesterone secretion with a basal production, which is independent from LH. Second, the large luteal cells, which derive from the theca cells, respond to LH with an increased progesterone and also estradiol production (Table 1) [9]. This can be found from 4 to 6 days after ovulation [10].

2.3 The Endometrium Under Hormonal Influences

It is well known that in every normal menstrual cycle, vascular and endometrial tissues undergo substantial proliferation processes in the "proliferative" phase which finds it ovarian counterpart in the follicular phase. From an endocrine perspective, the endometrium is estradiol-dominated in this phase. After ovulation and the formation of a corpus luteum, the endometrium enters the "secretory" phase, which is dominated by progesterone. If pregnancy does not occur, the demise of the corpus luteum leads to a decrease in progesterone levels and, thus, endometrial breakdown and shedding. With the beginning of the next endometrial cycle, i.e., the next proliferative phase, endometrial repair is started, which includes processes of angiogenesis, tissue remodeling, and formation of new tissue [10].

From a histological perspective, the endometrium consists of a simple columnar epithelium which overlies a multicellular stroma. In the stroma, fibroblast-like stromal cells, tubular glands adjacent to the luminal surface, spiral arteries, and innate

Table 1 Characteristics of small and large luteal cells [9]

Small luteal cells	Large luteal cells
Originate from granulosa cells	Originate from theca cells
Not responsive to LH	Responsive to LH (from 4 to 6 days after ovulation)
Produce autocrine and paracrine peptides and eicosanoids	Respond to LH pulses with increased production of estradiol and progesterone
Basal production of estradiol and progesterone	

immune cells can be found [10, 11]. Moreover, adult stem cells, so-called endometrial progenitor cells, have been described in the basal layer of the endometrium. These cells might have the capacity to differentiate into stromal and epithelial cells, thereby contributing to the repair processes after endometrial shedding [12].

Under the influence of progesterone, the endometrial stroma cells transform into decidual cells, which are secretory and provide a special microenvironment for embryo implantation and placentation. This transformation process is called "decidualization" [10, 13]. In the late secretory/luteal phase, together with the demise of luteal-phase follicular waves, progesterone contributes to the decline in circulating estradiol levels by promoting the conversion of estradiol to its less biologically active form estrone [14]. Moreover, the endometrial expression of the estrogen receptor is also reduced by progesterone [15]. Thereby, progesterone seems to lead to an overall inhibition of estradiol action [10].

If no pregnancy occurs, the withdrawal of progesterone and also estradiol leads to several morphological alterations of the endometrium, namely, tissue edema, increased endometrial blood flow, increased vessel permeability, and fragility [16–18]. In addition, large numbers of leukocytes can be found [19]. These processes ultimately lead to shedding of the so-called functional zone of the endometrium, i.e., the functional endometrial layer. In other words, menstruation occurs [10].

3 Luteal Phase Defects

3.1 General Pathophysiologic Considerations

Luteal phase defects (LPDs) were described for the first time in 1949 by Jones [20]. Originally, they were characterized by a failure to develop a fully mature endometrium [21]. This inadequate or out-of-phase transformation of the endometrium then can lead to problems in embryo implantation. From an etiologic perspective, LPDs can be due to an inadequate endometrial response to hormonal stimuli, first and foremost progesterone, or to an inadequate corpus luteum function. For the latter, several mechanisms have been proposed [21]:

- An insufficient LH surge
- An impaired luteotropic system
- Increased luteolysis
- Primary dysfunction of the corpus luteum

Various factors have been mentioned to be associated with LPDs, either at the level of the endometrium or of the corpus luteum, which are listed in Table 2. Figure 2 provides a schematic overview about pathophysiological principles involved.

Table 2 Factors associated with luteal phase defects

Decreased levels of FSH in follicular phase
Abnormal LH pulsatility in the luteal phase
Decreased levels of LH and FSH during the ovulatory surge
Elevated prolactin levels
Decreased response of the endometrium to progesterone
Inadequate expression of endometrial progesterone receptor
(Chronic) endometritis
Drug effects: clomiphene citrate, gonadotropin-releasing hormone (GnRH) agonists and antagonists

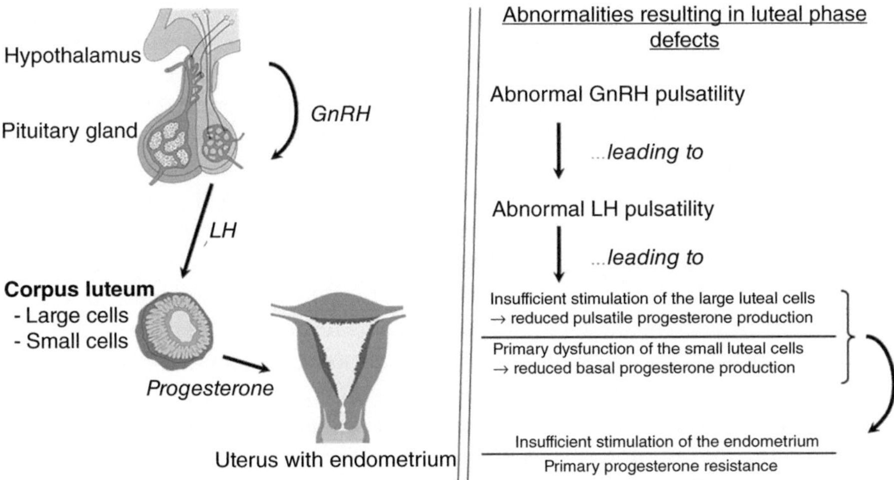

Fig. 2 Principle pathophysiologic processes involved in luteal phase defects

3.2 Diagnostic Considerations

LPDs are defined by a lag of more than 2 days in the histologic development of endometrium compared with the day of the cycle. In other words, the endometrial structure must be more than 2 days behind the expected day, defined by the preceding ovulation or the subsequent onset of menses. This situation must be present in more than one cycle due to the intercyclic variability [21].

Notably, a lag of 2 or more than 2 days behind the expected day of ovulation and the subsequent onset of menses, defined by the histologic dating method of Noyes et al. [22, 23], showed reproducibility to within 2 days of basal body temperature charts in more than 80% of the 8000 biopsy specimens which had been studied. Comparing the retrospective method with the day of ovulation as the reference point, 42% out-of-phase endometrium samples were found versus 10% using the prospective methods (reference point: next menstruation). Moreover, one must note that there is significant intra- and interobserver disagreement [24–26].

In addition to these uncertainties, the fact that more than one histological analyses are necessary per definition makes it hard to establish the diagnosis in clinical routine, especially in women who wish to conceive, where endometrial biopsy is not easily performed in the luteal phase.

Thus, several indicators have been evaluated in the past. To make it short, body temperature was found unreliable [21], which directly leads us to the considerations about the usefulness of progesterone measurements in serum. A problem in the small cells can be caused by accelerated luteolysis, and a problem in the large cells by a failure to respond to LH or a problem in the central regulation [9]. As stated above, progesterone levels also depend on GnRH-/LH-pulses from 4 to 6 days after the ovulation on. Thus, large fluctuations can be found which is due to the pulsatile release of GnRH [8]. With these circumstances in mind, it becomes evident that one single progesterone measurement carries a high risk of a false-negative or a false-positive result. To provide two examples, one could measure progesterone quite a long time after the last LH pulse, and, thus, a low progesterone level would be found. In consequence, one might suspect luteal deficiency. On the other hand, in a truly progesterone-deficient woman, one could derive one incorrectly normal result as well, if the sample is taking directly after one of the rare LH surges [8]. It has been estimated that one single progesterone measurement would lead to the false diagnosis of a luteal phase defect in about 15%. Thus, it has been suggested to take two or three samples within a period of 3 h with the aim of decreasing the probability of a false-positive result down to 2% and 0.5%, respectively (reviewed in [21]). It must be noted that all these progesterone measurements should be done 7 days after ovulation at the earliest to ensure that the complete function of the corpus luteum can be assessed, which means that it must already be responsive to LH [8].

Concerning the cut-off levels used for the diagnosis of a luteal phase defect, different progesterone levels have been reported (5 ng/mL, 8 ng/mL, 10 ng/mL) [21]. However, the highest accuracy was shown when a midluteal serum progesterone <10 ng/mL with a single measurement was used or <30 ng/mL as the sum of three random measurements [27].

Notably, neither luteal phase length nor the preovulatory maximum follicle diameter was found to be reliable alternatives to predict luteal phase defects. Thus, the serum progesterone level is the only relevant surrogate parameter [21].

3.3 The Clinical Relevance of Luteal Phase Defects

Concerning the clinical impact of classic luteal phase defects, the focus will be on three common entities: (i) infertility, especially unexplained infertility; (ii) luteal function after artificial reproduction, i.e., luteal support after in vitro fertilization (IVF); and (iii) recurrent miscarriage. Notably, it has been demonstrated that the rate of women with LPDs would be higher in infertility with about 12% and highest in recurrent miscarriage (up to 30%), when compared to fertile controls [28].

3.3.1 Luteal Phase Defects and Unexplained Infertility

It seems reasonable that the prevalence of LPDs would be higher in a population of women with unexplained infertility. However, several studies have demonstrated that the presence of an out-phase endometrium might not alter pregnancy chances. In 60 women treated with clomiphene-citrate, the pregnancy rate was 61.8% and 57.7% in women with and without histologically confirmed LPDs, respectively [29]. Similar findings were seen in women who had their endometrial biopsy in the cycle of conception [30]—a study which would be considerably difficult to conduct nowadays. Nonetheless, it could be demonstrated that the chances for pregnancy were associated with the severity of LPDs: pregnancy was more likely in women with less severe defects, and the mean endometrial lag time was 6.3 and 4.3 days ($p = 0.02$) in clomiphene-citrate treated women who became pregnant and those who did not, respectively [31].

Despite the remaining uncertainties about the impact of LPDs on fertility, evidence from frozen IVF cycles and donor cycles suggests that progesterone is of major impact. This assumption is based on the observation that in women without basal hormonal production, namely, women with hypogonadism, higher implantation rates could be achieved with the use of estradiol and progesterone supplementation compared to normally cycling women in some studies [32].

Given the fact that the benefit of luteal supplementation in women with unexplained infertility has not been finally proven, taken all the abovementioned considerations together, many physicians rely on pathogenesis-oriented treatments: estrogen and/or progesterone replacement, ovulation induction, luteal phase support with HCG, and lowering of prolactin levels when necessary. In clinical routine, many institutions offer clomiphene or letrozole stimulation or luteal phase support to couples with unexplained infertility despite the low evidence. However, more evidence is available from IVF cycles.

3.3.2 Luteal (Dys-)Function After IVF

Several possible pathophysiologic mechanisms for luteal dysfunction and LPDs in the course of IVF cycles have been proposed and are listed in Table 3 [33].

It has been clearly demonstrated that the use of luteal phase support with any kind of progestogen would increase the rates for ongoing pregnancy and live birth after IVF. However, as also shown in a Cochrane database analysis, this effect is

Table 3 Possible pathophysiologic mechanisms specific for IVF treatment, which could interfere with progesterone production and action on the endometrium

Multiple follicular development → supraphysiological levels of estradiol and progesterone → negative feedback on LH secretion
Prolonged suppression of the pituitary after administration of GnRH agonist or antagonist
Negative feedback of exogenous HCG on LH secretion

only modest with an odds ratio of about 1.8 [34]. This supports the often-mentioned theory that in the majority of patients who undergo fresh cycles, the natural luteal function is sufficient. It is well known that several routes for progesterone administration exist: intramuscular, vaginal, subcutaneous, oral, and transdermal [33]. An overview on commonly used regimen can be found in Table 4.

Fortunately, several good analyses which compared some of these schemes to each other are available. First, in a meta-analysis of 2009, the vaginal and the intramuscular applications were compared to each other. The effects on clinical and ongoing pregnancy were comparable, whereas the data favored the intravaginal progesterone in terms of a reduced miscarriage rate. It needs to be emphasized that a progesterone gel instead of capsules was used in that time [35]. In the last years, a discussion started whether oral dydrogesterone would be as effective as vaginal micronized progesterone. According to a meta-analysis in 2016, both regimens were similarly effective in terms of clinical pregnancy rate. However, the data favored oral dydrogesterone in terms of patient satisfaction [36]. Since the non-inferiority of oral dydrogesterone remained open, Griesinger and colleagues conducted the large, multicenter randomized "Lotus II"-study. Finally, the non-inferiority of oral dydrogesterone compared to vaginal progesterone could be demonstrated [37]. Table 5 provides an overview about the findings of the abovementioned studies.

In conclusion, although it is safe to say that the majority of preparations used seem to lead to similar conception and live birth rates, experts can rely on the existing data that oral application of dydrogesterone is reliable.

However, treatment with progesterone and dydrogesterone is not the only luteal support which has been tested. Notably, a meta-analysis showed favorable data for the use of HCG versus no luteal support with an odds ratio of 1.76 (95%CI: 1.08–2.86) for the combined outcome of ongoing pregnancy and live birth [34]. Several regimens of HCG dose have been used in the past, and it is unclear which one to favor. One commonly used regimen is the intramuscular application of 1500 international units on the day of oocyte retrieval and on 2, 4, and 6 days thereafter.

Estrogen + progesterone did not prove to be superior to progesterone only for luteal support in terms of clinical pregnancy rates and ongoing pregnancy rates/live birth [34]. However, last but not the least, since the production and secretion of progesterone are dependent on GnRH pulses [8, 9], it seems reasonable to also provide additional luteal support with GnRH-agonists. The already cited meta-analysis

Table 4 Commonly used regimen for luteal phase support with progesterone/gestagens after IVF

Intramuscular: oil based, 25–100 mg daily (standard: 50 mg)

Vaginal
  – Micronized vaginal progesterone bio-adhesive gel (Crinone® 8% 90 mg/day)
  – Vaginal progesterone capsules 200–400 mg daily
  – Vaginal ring (Milprosa®, weekly)
  – Subcutaneous: 25(−50) mg daily

Oral
  – Micronized progesterone in-oil capsules 600 mg/day
  – Dydrogesterone 10 mg 2–3/day

Table 5 Overview on relevant analyses comparing different routes of luteal support in IVF

	Type of analysis	Miscarriage rate	Clinical pregnancy rate	Ongoing pregnancy rate	Live birth rate
Progesterone versus no luteal support [34]	Meta-analysis	OR 0.54 [95%CI 0.29–1.02]*	OR 1.89 [95%CI 1.30–2.75]*	OR 1.77 [95%CI 1.09–2.86]*	
Vaginal versus intramuscular progesterone [35]	Meta-analysis	OR 0.54 [95%CI 0.29–1.02]*	OR 0.91 [95%CI 0.74–1.13]	OR 0.94 [95%CI 0.71–1.26]	–
Oral dydrogesterone versus vaginal micronized progesterone [36]	Meta-analysis	RR 0.77 [95%CI 0.53–1.10]	RR 1.07 [95%CI 0.93–1.23]	RR 1.04 [95%CI 0.92–1.18]	–
Oral dydrogesterone versus vaginal micronized progesterone [37]	RCT, non-inferiority analysis	–	–	AD 3.7% [95%CI −2.3–9.7]	AD 1.9% [95%CI −4.0–7.8]

OR odds ratio, *RR* risk ratio, *AD* adjusted difference, *95%CI* 95% confidence interval, *RCT* randomized controlled trial
*Statistically significant ($p < 0.05$)

from 2015 showed that progesterone only would be inferior to a GnRH-agonist + progesterone treatment (odds ratio 0.62, 95%CI 0.48–0.81) [34]. These data were confirmed by a more recent meta-analysis published in 2020 which clearly showed a beneficial effect of luteal support with a GnRH-agonist (live birth rate, relative risk 1.52; 95%CI, 1.20–1.94) [38].

However, in a natural ovulatory cycle, where LH supports the corpus luteum to secrete progesterone after ovulation, and in controlled ovarian hyperstimulation with an HCG trigger, where HCG mimics LH activity, the use of a GnRH-agonist trigger after controlled ovarian hyperstimulation might lead to worse luteal function. Notably, it is associated with a shorter luteal phase (9 versus 13 days) and decreased levels of progesterone and estradiol. Several strategies to overcome this negative effect have been proposed: the use of a dual trigger with low-dose HCG (1000–2500 IU) and GnRH-a, low-dose HCG (1500 IU) at the time of ovum pick-up, low-dose HCG in the luteal phase (1500 IU 3d after ovum pick-up or 125 IU daily), or more intensive luteal support (frequent monitoring: progesterone>20 ng/mL and estradiol>200 pg/mL) [33].

3.3.3 Luteal Phase Defects and Recurrent Miscarriage

There are various definitions for recurrent miscarriage. However, it is defined as the failure of a minimum of two clinically recognized pregnancies before 20–24 weeks of gestation [39]. As also mentioned above, LPDs seem quite common in women with recurrent miscarriage, with its prevalence ranging from about to 17% to nearly

30% [28, 40]. Particularly in cases of unexplained recurrent miscarriages, luteal phase defects are believed to be an important underlying cause.

It has been mentioned that low-dose stimulation might overcome the burden of histologically diagnosed luteal phase defects in these women in order to avoid insufficient FSH or LH levels in the follicular phase or around ovulation. According to one study, the use of low-dose stimulation with urinary-derived human menopausal gonadotropins was seemingly helpful [41]. However, the main approach is luteal phase support with progesterone/progestagens. Many studies have been published in the recent decades. This chapter will only focus on the currently relevant literature.

Notably, whether progesterone or gestagens should be used in women with recurrent miscarriage, especially unexplained recurrent miscarriage, is controversial. The use of gestagens in the first trimester has been investigated in a variety of studies. A meta-analysis, which included more than 1500 women with unexplained recurrent miscarriage and was published in 2017, revealed a beneficial effect on the rate of future pregnancy losses (RR 0.72, 95%CI 0.53–0.97) and of live births (RR 1.07, 95%CI 1.02–1.15). However, these results were significant only for synthetic gestagens rather than micronized progesterone [42]. A similar but more recent meta-analysis revealed a similar findings, namely, that in unexplained recurrent miscarriages, supplementation with progestogen therapy may reduce the rate of miscarriage in subsequent pregnancies (RR 0.73, 95CI 0.54–1.00, moderate-quality evidence) and may increase the chance for a future live birth (RR 1.07, 95%CI 1.00–1.13, moderate-quality evidence) [43].

The largest available single study is the PROMISE trial. Noteworthy, in this long awaited study, two vaginal capsules of 200 mg micronized progesterone did not lead to a beneficial effect in women with unexplained recurrent miscarriage. In detail, the live birth rates were 65.8% (262/398) and 63.3% (271/428) in the progesterone and the placebo groups, respectively (RR 1.04, 95%CI 0.94–1.15; $p = 0.45$) [44]. In a second analysis of both the PROMISE and the PRISM studies, vaginal progesterone treatment as indicated above was beneficial for women with threatened miscarriage and three or more previous early miscarriages [45]. The most recent Cochrane database network meta-analysis revealed similar results: vaginal micronized progesterone (RR 1.03, 95%CI 1.00–1.07) and dydrogesterone (RR 0.98, 95%CI 0.89–1.07) were judged as "probably making little or no difference to the live birth rate when compared with placebo for women with threatened miscarriage" [46]. It should be noted that the modest effect size might be explained by the fact that an inadequate secretion of the corpus luteum might not so much be the cause of a disturbed early pregnancy, but rather the consequence of a restricted embryonic development with subsequent insufficient HCG levels and lack of stimulation of the corpus luteum.

However, in women with no previous miscarriages and early pregnancy bleeding, no improvement in the live birth rate was found with vaginal micronized progesterone compared to placebo (RR 0.99, 95%CI 0.95–1.04). However, for women with one or more previous miscarriages and early pregnancy bleeding, vaginal micronized progesterone increased the live birth rate compared to placebo (RR

1.08, 95%CI 1.02–1.15) [46]. It can be concluded from this evidence that women with unexplained recurrent miscarriage can be treated with natural micronized progesterone and that women with unexplained recurrent miscarriage and threatened miscarriage should be vaginally treated with natural micronized progesterone, which is in line with current guidelines as the AWMF guideline (available online https://www.awmf.org/leitlinien/detail/ll/015-050.html).

4 Endometrial Function in Polycystic Ovary Syndrome: A Special Situation

An altered endometrial function in polycystic ovary syndrome (PCOS) is obvious, since PCOS women reveal an increased risk for endometrial cancer, implantation failure, pregnancy complications, and possibly miscarriage/recurrent miscarriage [47]. Given the high worldwide prevalence of PCOS, which ranges from 4% to 21% and depends on the diagnostic criteria used [48], it has been suggested that altered endometrial function in PCOS is likely due to primary abnormalities ("prenatal programming") as well as secondary abnormalities ("postnatal alterations"). The first include aberrant expression of sex hormone receptors and their co-regulators, aberrant expression of gene regulation, various cell processes, and abnormal regulation of enzymatic and metabolic pathways, whereas the latter include the well-known pathophysiologic processes of PCOS, namely, high estrogen/low progesterone levels due to oligo-/anovulation, insulin resistance, and chronic low-grade inflammation. Details about these mechanisms are perfectly summed up in the recent review by Palomba et al. [47].

4.1 PCOS and Endometrial Cancer

Without a doubt, the risk for endometrial cancer is increased in women with PCOS. In a meta-analysis, an OR of 2.79 (95%CI (CI), 1.31–5.95; $p < 0.008$) was found. Notably, the risk seems to be even higher in premenopausal women (PCOS patients <54 years, OR 4.05, 95%CI: 2.42–6.76, $p < 0.001$) [48]. This increase in risk is independent from known other risk factors which also include obesity [47, 49]. Notably, it is unclear whether primary or secondary abnormalities or both are responsible. Moreover, it has not been clarified, whether the basic risk, which is independent from general risk factors, can be modified. The only preventive measure is the pragmatic approach of bleeding induction with combined oral contraception or progestin therapy, since the optimal prevention for endometrial hyperplasia and endometrial cancer is unknown, which has been recommended by the International PCOS network in 2018 [50].

4.2 Progesterone Resistance in PCOS

The actions of progesterone on the endometrium include downregulation of the estrogen receptor, upregulation of enzymes involved in estrogen metabolization, restriction of androgen receptor expression, and the downregulation of its own receptors [10, 51]. In women with PCOS, an imbalance between progesterone levels/action and estrogen levels/action is likely due to chronic oligo-/anovulation and also a PCOS-specific progesterone resistance [47]. The existence of the latter is highly suggested by its systemic appearance, since progesterone resistance has also been described at the pituitary level [52, 53]. Hypothetically, an increased androgen receptor expression might be the cause [54, 55] as well as an altered gene expression of progesterone receptor isoforms [56, 57]. These assumptions lead to the question, whether women with PCOS would benefit from progestin/progesterone treatment in the case of infertility and/or ovarian stimulation for oligo-/anovulation. Notably, conventional doses of progesterone were not enough to correct the changes of endometrial histomorphology and specific endometrial markers completely [58].

4.3 Clinical Considerations

4.3.1 Letrozole, Clomiphene Citrate, and Low-Dose FSH Stimulation

Concerning ovarian stimulation in PCOS women, one has to consider two major questions about the use of progestins/progesterone: (i) is the induction of endometrial shedding prior to ovarian stimulation beneficial in terms of pregnancy rates, and (ii) is luteal support after ovulation induction necessary? Despite the high prevalence of PCOS, literature on these issues is scarce.

In a secondary analysis of a randomized, double-blinded study about clomiphene citrate with or without metformin in PCOS patients, it could be shown that endometrial shedding, either spontaneous or progestin-induced, prior to ovarian stimulation resulted in a reduction in the subsequent rate of conception and live birth (live birth per cycle, spontaneous menses 2.2%, anovulatory with progestin withdrawal 1.6%, anovulatory without progestin withdrawal 5.3%; $p < 0.001$; live birth per ovulation, spontaneous menses 3.0%, anovulatory with progestin withdrawal 5.4%, anovulatory without progestin withdrawal 19.7%; $p < 0.001$) [59]. Unfortunately, no data exist about stimulation with letrozole, which is the first-line stimulation agent for PCOS women [50]. One study showed that endometrial shedding induced by progesterone withdrawal did not negatively affect pregnancy rates in PCOS women undergoing letrozole stimulation and intrauterine insemination. However, the control group consisted of patients with spontaneous menses, and, thus, no women without endometrial shedding were included [60].

The second possible intervention for improvement of endometrial function would be luteal phase support. In a retrospective cohort study on women with PCOS who underwent ovarian stimulation with clomiphene citrate or letrozole, the pregnancy rate was seemingly higher when luteal phase support with intravaginal progesterone had been provided (27/162 cycles, 16.7% versus 11/104 cycles, 10.6%; $p > 0.05$). In letrozole cycles, clinical pregnancies were achieved in 21.1% of cycles (8/38) in the progesterone group, compared with none (0/13) in the non-progesterone group. Despite the fact that these results did not reach statistical significance, the authors concluded that "luteal supplementation with progesterone should be strongly considered in women with PCOS, especially in those using letrozole for ovulation induction" [61]. Comparable results were found in a randomized study on 110 clomiphene citrate-resistant PCOS patients, who underwent low-dose stimulation with recombinant FSH and intrauterine insemination. Luteal-supported cycles demonstrated a 6.7% higher clinical pregnancy rate and 6.1% higher live birth rate ($p > 0.05$) [62]. Given the paucity of data, no conclusion can be drawn about the usefulness of luteal support after clomiphene citrate, letrozole, and low-dose FSH stimulation in PCOS women, since larger randomized studies are necessary. However, from a practical point of view, to provide luteal support to these women seems reasonable.

4.3.2   IVF, PCOS, and Endometrial Function

One important intervention for improvement of endometrial function in PCOS patients who undergo IVF is elective frozen-thawed embryo transfer. This measure is based on the rationale to avoid endometrial dysfunction due to estrogen overload, which is highly likely in PCOS patients who are at an increased risk for polyfollicular development and ovarian hyperstimulation syndrome [63].

It has been postulated that supraphysiological estradiol exposure after ovarian hyperstimulation might lead to a disruption of embryo implantation after fresh embryo transfer. Thus, elective frozen embryo transfer might lead to favorable outcomes [64]. Although an initial prospective study, which randomized women who underwent their first IVF cycle to fresh embryo transfer versus elective frozen embryo transfer, showed only a significant reduction in the risk for ovarian hyperstimulation syndrome but no increase in the chance for a live birth [64], a secondary analysis of data from two multicenter randomized trials demonstrated that women with PCOS would benefit from elective frozen embryo transfer in terms of live birth rates when the peak estradiol level exceeded 3000 pg/mL (OR 1.57; 95%CI 1.22–2.03) or 16 oocytes were retrieved (OR 1.67; 95%CI 1.20–2.31) [63].

5   Conclusions

Although it has been asked whether luteal phase defects would only be a myth, it can be safely concluded that they exist and are of clinical impact on our patients. Per definition, luteal phase defects are characterized by a time lag in endometrial development [21]. Both dysfunction of the corpus luteum and decreased response of the endometrium to progesterone might be responsible. Despite the fact that many underlying pathophysiologic pathways have been blamed to be associated with luteal phase defects and its possible consequences, namely, infertility, recurrent implantation failure, and (recurrent) miscarriage, the majority of evidence deals with luteal support with gestagens. The support with vaginal micronized progesterone and, in the course of IVF, oral dydrogesterone is the most evidence-based measure. In addition, luteal support with HCG or GnRH analogues after IVF embryo transfer and the use of elective frozen embryo transfer in PCOS women with high peak estradiol have been demonstrated to increase the chance for ongoing pregnancy and/or live birth.

References

 1. Kol S. Time, time, time: see what governs the luteal phase endocrinology. Gynecol Endocrinol. 2021;37(9):775–7.
 2. Pache T, Wladimiroff J, DeJong F, Hop W, Fauser B. Growth patterns of nondominant ovarian follicles during the normal menstrual cycle. Fertil Steril. 1990;54:638–342.
 3. Hodgen G. The dominant ovarian follicle. Fertil Steril. 1982;38:281–300.
 4. McNatty KP, Hillier SG, Boogaard AMVD, Trimbos-Kemper TC, Reichert LK, Hall EVV. Follicular development during the luteal phase of the human menstrual cycle. J Clin Endocrinol Metab. 1983;56:1022–31.
 5. Baerwald AR, Adams GP, Pierson RA. Characterization of ovarian follicular wave dynamics in women. Biol Reprod. 2003;69(3):1023–31. https://doi.org/10.1095/biolreprod.103.017772.
 6. Baerwald AR, Adams GP, Pierson RA. A new model for ovarian follicular development during the human menstrual cycle. Fertil Steril. 2003;80(1):116–22.
 7. Vanden Brink H, Robertson DM, Lim H, Lee C, Chizen D, Harris G, Hale G, Burger H, Baerwald A. Associations between antral ovarian follicle dynamics and hormone production throughout the menstrual cycle as women age. J Clin Endocrinol Metab. 2015;100(12):4553–62.
 8. Wuttke W, Pitzel L, Seidlová-Wuttke D, Hinney B. LH pulses and the corpus luteum: the luteal phase deficiency LPD. Vitam Horm. 2001;63:131–58.
 9. Ohara A, Mori T, Taii S, Ban C, Narimoto K. Functional differentiation in steroidogenesis of two types of luteal cells isolated from mature human corpora lutea of menstrual cycle. J Clin Endocrinol Metab. 1987;65(6):1192–200.
10. Critchley HOD, Maybin JA, Armstrong GM, Williams ARW. Physiology of the endometrium and regulation of menstruation. Physiol Rev. 2020;100(3):1149–79.
11. Noyes RW, Hertig AT, Rock J. Dating the endometrial biopsy. Fertil Steril. 1950;1(1921):3–25.
12. Gargett CE, Masuda H. Adult stem cells in the endometrium. Mol Hum Reprod. 2010;16(11):818–34.
13. Gellersen B, Brosens JJ. Cyclic decidualization of the human endometrium in reproductive health and failure. Endocr Rev. 2014;35(6):851–905.
14. Tseng L, Gurpide E. Estradiol and 20alpha-dihydroprogesterone dehydrogenase activities in human endometrium during the menstrual cycle. Endocrinology. 1974;94:419–23.
15. Tseng L, Gurpide E. Effects of progestins on estradiol receptor levels in human endometrium. J Clin Endocrinol Metab. 1975;41:402–4.
16. Garry R, Hart R, Karthigasu KA, Burke C. Structural changes in endometrial basal glands during menstruation. BJOG. 2010;117:1175–85.

17. Finn CA. Implantation, menstruation and inflammation. Biol Rev Camb Philos Soc. 1986;61:313–28.
18. Roberts DK, Parmley TH, Walker NJ, Horbelt DV. Ultrastructure of the microvasculature in the human endometrium throughout the normal menstrual cycle. Am J Obstet Gynecol. 1992;166:1393–406.
19. Evans J, Salamonsen LA. Inflammation, leukocytes and menstruation. Rev Endocr Metab Disord. 2012;13:277–88.
20. Jones GES. Some newer aspects of the management of infertility. JAMA. 1949;141:1123–9.
21. Bukulmez O, Arici A. Luteal phase defect: myth or reality. Obstet Gynecol Clin N Am. 2004;31(4):727–44.
22. Noyes RW, Hertig MD, Rock MD. Dating the endometrial biopsy. Fertil Steril. 1950;1950(1):3–25.
23. Noyes RW, Hamano JO. Accuracy of endometrial dating, correlation of endometrial dating with basal body temperature and menses. Fertil Steril. 1953;4(6):504–17.
24. Jones GS, Madrigal-Castro V. Hormonal findings in association with abnormal corpus luteum function in the human: the luteal phase defect. Fertil Steril. 1970;21(1):1–13.
25. Balasch J, Vanrell JA, Creus M, Marquez M, Gonzalez-Merlo J. The endometrial biopsy for diagnosis of luteal phase deficiency. Fertil Steril. 1985;44(5):699–701.
26. Li TC, Rogers AW, Lenton EA, Dockery P, Cooke I. A comparison between two methods of chronological dating of human endometrial biopsies during the luteal phase, and their correlation with histologic dating. Fertil Steril. 1987;48(6):928–32.
27. Jordan J, Craig K, Clifton DK, Soules MR. Luteal phase defect: the sensitivity and specificity of diagnostic methods in common clinical use. Fertil Steril. 1994;62(1):54–62.
28. Balasch J, Creus M, Márquez M, Burzaco I, Vanrell JA. The significance of luteal phase deficiency on fertility: a diagnostic and therapeutic approach. Hum Reprod. 1986;1(3):145–7.
29. Wentz AC, Kossoy LR, Parker RA. The impact of luteal phase inadequacy in an infertile population. Am J Obstet Gynecol. 1990;162(4):937–45.
30. Balasch J, Fábregues F, Creus M, Vanrell JA. The usefulness of endometrial biopsy for luteal phase evaluation in infertility. Hum Reprod. 1992;7(7):973–7.
31. Downs KA, Gibson M. Clomiphene citrate therapy for luteal phase defect. Fertil Steril. 1983;39(1):34–8.
32. Edwards RG, Morcos S, Macnamee M, Balmaceda JP, Walters DE, Asch R. High fecundity of amenorrhoeic women in embryo-transfer programmes. Lancet. 1991;338(8762):292–4.
33. Dashti S, Eftekhar M. Luteal-phase support in assisted reproductive technology: an ongoing challenge. Int J Reprod Biomed. 2021;19(9):761–72.
34. van der Linden M, Buckingham K, Farquhar C, Kremer JA, Metwally M. Luteal phase support for assisted reproduction cycles. Cochrane Database Syst Rev. 2015;(7):CD009154.
35. Zarutskie PW, Phillips JA. A meta-analysis of the route of administration of luteal phase support in assisted reproductive technology: vaginal versus intramuscular progesterone. Fertil Steril. 2009;92(1):163–9.
36. Barbosa MW, Silva LR, Navarro PA, Ferriani RA, Nastri CO, Martins WP. Dydrogesterone vs progesterone for luteal-phase support: systematic review and meta-analysis of randomized controlled trials. Ultrasound Obstet Gynecol. 2016;48(2):161–70.
37. Griesinger G, Blockeel C, Sukhikh GT, Patki A, Dhorepatil B, Yang DZ, Chen ZJ, Kahler E, Pexman-Fieth C, Tournaye H. Oral dydrogesterone versus intravaginal micronized progesterone gel for luteal phase support in IVF: a randomized clinical trial. Hum Reprod. 2018;33(12):2212–21.
38. Ma X, Du W, Hu J, Yang Y, Zhang X. Effect of gonadotrophin-releasing hormone agonist addition for luteal support on pregnancy outcome in vitro fertilization/intracytoplasmic sperm injection cycles: a meta-analysis based on randomized controlled trials. Gynecol Obstet Investig. 2020;85(1):13–25.
39. Dimitriadis E, Menkhorst E, Saito S, Kutteh WH, Brosens JJ. Recurrent pregnancy loss. Nat Rev Dis Primers. 2020;6(1):98.

40. Li TC. Recurrent miscarriage: principles of management. Hum Reprod. 1998;13(2):478–82.
41. Li TC, Ding SH, Anstie B, Tuckerman E, Wood K, Laird S. Use of human menopausal gonadotropins in the treatment of endometrial defects associated with recurrent miscarriage: preliminary report. Fertil Steril. 2001;75(2):434–7.
42. Saccone G, Schoen C, Franasiak JM, Scott RT Jr, Berghella V. Supplementation with progestogens in the first trimester of pregnancy to prevent miscarriage in women with unexplained recurrent miscarriage: a systematic review and meta-analysis of randomized, controlled trials. Fertil Steril. 2017;107(2):430–8.
43. Haas DM, Hathaway TJ, Ramsey PS. Progestogen for preventing miscarriage in women with recurrent miscarriage of unclear etiology. Cochrane Database Syst Rev. 2019;(11):CD003511.
44. Coomarasamy A, Williams H, Truchanowicz E, Seed PT, Small R, Quenby S, Gupta P, Dawood F, Koot YE, Atik RB, Bloemenkamp KW, Brady R, Briley A, Cavallaro R, Cheong YC, Chu J, Eapen A, Essex H, Ewies A, Hoek A, Kaaijk EM, Koks CA, Li TC, MacLean M, Mol BW, Moore J, Parrott S, Ross JA, Sharpe L, Stewart J, Trépel D, Vaithilingam N, Farquharson RG, Kilby MD, Khalaf Y, Goddijn M, Regan L, Rai R. PROMISE: first-trimester progesterone therapy in women with a history of unexplained recurrent miscarriages—a randomised, double-blind, placebo-controlled, international multicentre trial and economic evaluation. Health Technol Assess. 2016;20(41):1–92.
45. Coomarasamy A, Devall AJ, Brosens JJ, Quenby S, Stephenson MD, Sierra S, Christiansen OB, Small R, Brewin J, Roberts TE, Dhillon-Smith R, Harb H, Noordali H, Papadopoulou A, Eapen A, Prior M, Di Renzo GC, Hinshaw K, Mol BW, Lumsden MA, Khalaf Y, Shennan A, Goddijn M, van Wely M, Al-Memar M, Bennett P, Bourne T, Rai R, Regan L, Gallos ID. Micronized vaginal progesterone to prevent miscarriage: a critical evaluation of randomized evidence. Am J Obstet Gynecol. 2020;223(2):167–76.
46. Devall AJ, Papadopoulou A, Podesek M, Haas DM, Price MJ, Coomarasamy A, Gallos ID. Progestogens for preventing miscarriage: a network meta-analysis. Cochrane Database Syst Rev. 2021;4(4):CD013792.
47. Palomba S, Piltonen TT, Giudice LC. Endometrial function in women with polycystic ovary syndrome: a comprehensive review. Hum Reprod Update. 2021;27(3):584–618.
48. Lizneva D, Suturina L, Walker W, Brakta S, Gavrilova-Jordan L, Azziz R. Criteria, prevalence, and phenotypes of polycystic ovary syndrome. Fertil Steril. 2016;106(1):6–15.
49. Barry JA, Azizia MM, Hardiman PJ. Risk of endometrial, ovarian and breast cancer in women with polycystic ovary syndrome: a systematic review and meta-analysis. Hum Reprod Update. 2014;20(5):748–58.
50. Teede HJ, Misso ML, Costello MF, Dokras A, Laven J, Moran L, Piltonen T, Norman RJ. International PCOS network recommendations from the international evidence-based guideline for the assessment and management of polycystic ovary syndrome. Fertil Steril. 2018;110(3):364–79.
51. MacLaughlan SD, Palomino WA, Mo B, Lewis TD, Lininger RA, Lessey BA. Endometrial expression of Cyr61: a marker of estrogenic activity in normal and abnormal endometrium. Obstet Gynecol. 2007;110(1):146–54.
52. Daniels TL, Berga SL. Resistance of gonadotropin releasing hormone drive to sex steroid-induced suppression in hyperandrogenic anovulation. J Clin Endocrinol Metab. 1997;82(12):4179–83.
53. Pastor CL, Griffin-Korf ML, Aloi JA, Evans WS, Marshall JC. Polycystic ovary syndrome: evidence for reduced sensitivity of the gonadotropin-releasing hormone pulse generator to inhibition by estradiol and progesterone. J Clin Endocrinol Metab. 1998;83(2):582–90.
54. Slayden OD, Brenner RM. Flutamide counteracts the antiproliferative effects of antiprogestins in the primate endometrium. J Clin Endocrinol Metab. 2003;88(2):946–9.
55. Slayden OD, Nayak NR, Burton KA, Chwalisz K, Cameron ST, Critchley HO, Baird DT, Brenner RM. Progesterone antagonists increase androgen receptor expression in the rhesus macaque and human endometrium. J Clin Endocrinol Metab. 2001;86(6):2668–79.

56. Patel B, Elguero S, Thakore S, Dahoud W, Bedaiwy M, Mesiano S. Role of nuclear progesterone receptor isoforms in uterine pathophysiology. Hum Reprod Update. 2015;21(2):155–73.
57. Li X, Feng Y, Lin JF, Billig H, Shao R. Endometrial progesterone resistance and PCOS. J Biomed Sci. 2014;21(1):2.
58. Lopes IM, Maganhin CC, Oliveira-Filho RM, Simões RS, Simões MJ, Iwata MC, Baracat EC, Soares JM Jr. Histomorphometric analysis and markers of endometrial receptivity embryonic implantation in women with polycystic ovary syndrome during the treatment with progesterone. Reprod Sci. 2014;21(7):930–8.
59. Diamond MP, Kruger M, Santoro N, Zhang H, Casson P, Schlaff W, Coutifaris C, Brzyski R, Christman G, Carr BR, McGovern PG, Cataldo NA, Steinkampf MP, Gosman GG, Nestler JE, Carson S, Myers EE, Eisenberg E, Legro RS, Eunice Kennedy Shriver National Institute of Child Health and Human Development Cooperative Reproductive Medicine Network. Endometrial shedding effect on conception and live birth in women with polycystic ovary syndrome. Obstet Gynecol. 2012;119(5):902–8.
60. Dong X, Zheng Y, Liao X, Xiong T, Zhang H. Does progesterone-induced endometrial withdrawal bleed before ovulation induction have negative effects on IUI outcomes in patients with polycystic ovary syndrome? Int J Clin Exp Pathol. 2013;6(6):1157–63.
61. Montville CP, Khabbaz M, Aubuchon M, Williams DB, Thomas MA. Luteal support with intravaginal progesterone increases clinical pregnancy rates in women with polycystic ovary syndrome using letrozole for ovulation induction. Fertil Steril. 2010;94(2):678–83.
62. Yazici G, Savas A, Tasdelen B, Dilek S. Role of luteal phase support on gonadotropin ovulation induction cycles in patients with polycystic ovary syndrome. J Reprod Med. 2014;59(1–2):25–30.
63. Kollmann M, Martins WP, Lima ML, Craciunas L, Nastri CO, Richardson A, Raine-Fenning N. Strategies for improving outcome of assisted reproduction in women with polycystic ovary syndrome: systematic review and meta-analysis. Ultrasound Obstet Gynecol. 2016;48(6):709–18.
64. Wei D, Yu Y, Sun M, Shi Y, Sun Y, Deng X, Li J, Wang Z, Zhao S, Zhang H, Legro RS, Chen ZJ. The effect of supraphysiological estradiol on pregnancy outcomes differs between women with PCOS and ovulatory women. J Clin Endocrinol Metab. 2018;103(7):2735–42.

Management of Severe Premenstrual Syndrome (PMS)/Premenstrual Dysphoric Disorder (PMDD)

Nick Panay

1   Introduction, Definitions, and Guidelines

Premenstrual syndrome (PMS) has been defined as a condition which causes distressing physical, behavioral, and psychological symptoms, in the absence of organic or underlying psychiatric disease, which regularly recurs during the luteal phase of each menstrual cycle and which disappears or significantly regresses by the end of menstruation [1]. Almost 95% of women will experience mild physiological symptoms prior to menstruation; however around 5–8% experience severe symptoms such that they cause considerable disruption to their lives [2].

A form of severe PMS has been termed premenstrual dysphoric disorder (PMDD) by the American Psychiatric Association, originally in their DSM-IV classification, and has strict diagnostic criteria [3]. Over the course of a year, during most menstrual cycles, five or more key symptoms must be present. The symptoms must disturb ability to work socially or professionally, and symptoms must not be related to or exaggerated by another medical condition.

NAPS recently changed its name to the National Association for Premenstrual Syndromes from "…Syndrome" to reflect the variation in definitions and severities of this disorder. The author and NAPS believe that current PMS terminology should be maintained because PMDD refers to only one type of severe form of PMS.

One of the most accurate and comprehensive classification systems was proposed by the International Society for Premenstrual Disorders [4–5] as shown below.

N. Panay (✉)
Imperial College Healthcare NHS Trust, London, UK

Imperial College, London, UK

Beijing Obstetrics and Gynecology Hospital, Capital Medical University, Beijing, China

    95
A. R. Genazzani et al. (eds.), *Menstrual Bleeding and Pain Disorders from Adolescence to Menopause*, ISGE Series,
https://doi.org/10.1007/978-3-031-55300-4_8

Core premenstrual disorders (core PMD) are the most commonly encountered and widely recognized type of PMS. They must be present during the luteal phase and abate as menstruation begins, which is followed by a symptom-free week.

There are also PMDs that do not meet the criteria for core PMDs. These are called "variant" PMDs and fall into four subtypes:

1. *Premenstrual exacerbation of an underlying disorder,* such as diabetes, depression, epilepsy, asthma, and migraine.
2. *Non-ovulatory premenstrual disorders* occur in the presence of ovarian activity without ovulation.
3. *Progestogen-induced premenstrual disorders* are caused by exogenous progestogens present in hormone replacement therapy (HRT) and the combined oral contraceptive pill.
4. *Premenstrual disorders without menstruation* include women who have a functioning ovarian cycle, but, for reasons such as hysterectomy, ablation, or the levonorgestrel intrauterine system, they do not menstruate.

Education of public and HCPs is the key issue going forward. It is vital that there is universal recognition of the severe impact that PMS can have, *whatever terminology is used.*

One of the most comprehensive set of evidence-based guidelines for managing this condition has been developed by the Royal College of Obstetricians and Gynaecologists [6]. These are a very useful tool for healthcare professionals to understand and manage this condition effectively. A recent review paper has been published which updates some of the information in the guideline and is a good state-of-the-art comprehensive review [7].

Other good sources of information for both the public and healthcare professionals are the websites of NAPS pms.org.uk and the International Association for Premenstrual Disorders IAPMD.org (see full links at the end of chapter).

2 Etiology

The etiology of PMS/PMDD remains poorly understood. The absence of PMS/PMDD before puberty, during pregnancy, and after the menopause highlights the role of cyclical ovarian activity in its pathogenesis.

Women with PMS/PMDD appear to produce the same levels of gonadal hormones as women without PMS/PMDD, and therefore it has been suggested that PMS/PMDD may be due to a differential sensitivity to circulating hormone metabolites rather than abnormal hormone levels [8].

Research appears to confirm this hypothesis in which estrogen receptor alpha gene polymorphisms have been found to differ in PMDD sufferers compared to controls [9]. Professor Goldman who led the research stated, "This is a big moment for women's health, because it establishes that women with PMDD have an intrinsic difference in their molecular apparatus for response to sex hormones – not just emotional behaviors they should be able to voluntarily control."

The ESC/E (Z) complex, an effector of response to ovarian steroids, has also been found to have intrinsic differences in cells from women with premenstrual dysphoric disorder [10].

The neurotransmitters serotonin and gamma-aminobutyric acid (GABA) have also been implicated as potential pathways through which abnormal responses to hormone levels may occur [11–12].

The late Professor John Studd, one of the great pioneers in this field, referred to "The triad of estrogen responsive depressive disorders in the same predisposed individual who would typically suffer with PMS/PMDD, postnatal depression and climacteric depression [13]." This individual typically feels well during the latter half of pregnancy when hormone levels are high and stable and does not experience symptoms pre pubertally and post menopausally.

3   Assessment and Diagnosis

Accurate prompt diagnosis of PMS/PMDD is essential in the effective management of this condition. A careful history should be sought, specifically for the cyclical nature of the symptoms. Premenstrual symptoms may commence up to 2 weeks prior to menstruation and resolve by the end of menstruation. To make the diagnosis, there should be a symptom-free interval prior to ovulation; however this may often be complicated by physical or psychiatric comorbidities. Premenstrual exacerbation of these conditions is now referred to as PME rather than PMDD.

Ideally symptoms should be assessed prospectively using symptom diaries over at least 2 consecutive months. Example symptom diaries can be found at https://pms.org.uk. Alternatively, menstrual cycle apps such as Flo and Clue can be used. In research, questionnaires such as the Daily Record of Severity of Problems (DRSP) are often used.

PMS/PMDD can cause a wide range of psychological, behavioral, and physical symptoms (see Table 1). In severe PMS/PMDD, some form of functional impairment, such as an inability to interact socially or professionally, will be evident.

Table 1 Symptoms associated with PMS

Psychological	Behavioral	Physical
Mood swings	Withdrawal	Bloating
Tearfulness	Lack of control	Pelvic pain
Irritability	Reduced concentration/cognitive ability	Breast tenderness
Depression	Poor sleep	Headaches
Anxiety		Food cravings
		Lethargy
		Weight gain

Any underlying conditions as suggested by the history should be excluded and managed appropriately. Common conditions which may cause diagnostic confusion include bipolar depressive disorder, generalized anxiety disorder, stress, polycystic ovarian syndrome, hypothyroidism, and alcohol or drug abuse. There appears to be an increasing preponderance of women with background ADHD or personality disorder and a history of abuse in childhood.

4 Management

Once the diagnosis has been confirmed, several management options are available, many of which can be used in the primary care setting. Treatments used are often unlicensed for the indication; however their use is justified when they are of proven efficacy and safety. As previously mentioned, the RCOG, NAPS, and IAPMD have published evidence-based treatment guidelines for PMS/PMDD which can be followed and are a useful "toolkit."

A potential treatment strategy for PMS/PMDD is shown in Fig. 1 which has been adopted by many guidelines.

4.1 Dietary and Lifestyle Approaches

All women should be given dietary and lifestyle advice on measures which may help reduce symptoms. The prevalence of PMS is increased in obese women and those who take less exercise. Weight loss and exercise have been shown to reduce

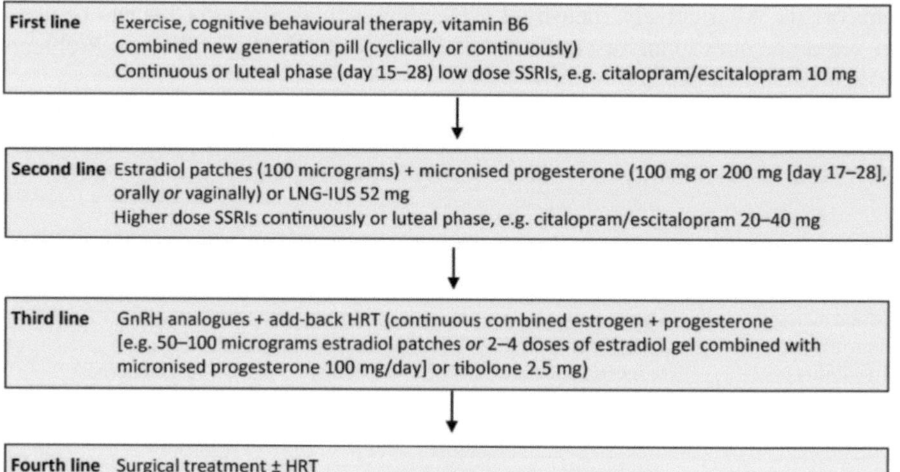

Fig. 1 Pragmatic management strategy for PMS/PMDD

PMS symptoms [14] and therefore should be recommended. Stress reduction and low glycemic index diets are also likely to be beneficial although no studies have examined these measures directly. Cognitive behavioral therapy has been shown to improve PMS symptoms and should be considered in all women [15]. NAPS and IAPMD can provide further support for sufferers although all healthcare professionals should be able to provide some help and signposting if adequately trained. Women with underlying psychopathology should be co-managed with a psychologist and/or psychiatrist.

4.2   Complementary Therapies

Some women may choose to use complementary therapies to manage their symptoms. There is some evidence to support the use of calcium and vitamin D, magnesium, or St. John's wort; however data for most complementary therapies remains inadequate, and the quality control of preparations cannot always be guaranteed [6–7]. A large placebo effect is generally observed, and women should be advised that there is the potential for side effects and drug interaction. The most evidence based of the complementary therapies for PMS/PMDD appears to be *Vitex agnus-castus* (VAC). In a recent meta-analysis, women taking VAC were 2.57 (95% CI 1.52–4.35) times more likely to experience a remission in their symptoms compared to those taking the placebo. However, as with most complementary therapies, many of the studies were small, and there was incomplete reporting of the types of preparations used [16].

4.3   Anti-depressants

Serotonin has been implicated in the pathogenesis of PMS/PMDD and is thought to be associated with symptoms such as irritability and low mood. Selective serotonin reuptake inhibitors (SSRIs) have been used for many years in the management. A meta- analysis has shown SSRIs (fluoxetine, paroxetine, sertraline, citalopram) are effective in reducing premenstrual symptoms in moderate or severe PMS [17]. They have been shown to reduce physical, functional, and behavioral premenstrual symptoms and improve quality of life [17]. SSRIs can be given either continuously or in the luteal phase only (i.e., days 15–28); both regimens appear to be of similar efficacy. The advantages of luteal phase treatment include avoidance of dependency and that the regimen is often more acceptable to women concerned about the stigma of using treatments usually associated with psychiatric conditions [17]. Some data also exist to support the use of the SNRI venlafaxine [18]; however further large-scale studies are needed.

4.4 Hormonal Treatment

Hormonal treatment in PMS/PMDD aims to suppress ovulation and stabilize hormonal fluctuations throughout the menstrual cycle.

4.4.1 Combined Oral Contraceptive Pill (COCP)

There is increasing evidence that new-generation COCPs are effective at reducing PMS/PMDD symptoms. The progesterone component of the COCP has been held responsible for the failure of older COCPs to improve PMS/PMDD, as a common side effect of progestogens is PMS-like symptoms. It is also thought that a standard 7-day hormone-free interval allows for follicular activity and therefore symptoms to resurge during that time.

The progestogen drospironone, contained in some COCP regimens, has anti-mineralocorticoid and anti-androgenic properties, which may help avoid progestogenic side effects such as bloating and irritability. The benefit of these regimens over placebo has been demonstrated for PMS/PMDD symptoms in a small randomized trial [19]; however convincing, large-scale data are lacking.

A further advance has been the development of lower-dose 20 mcg (rather than 30 mcg) ethinylestradiol COCPs containing drospironone, but in a 24/4 regimen, in contrast to the traditional 21/7 regimens. The shorter hormone-free interval is associated with more profound follicular suppression and more stable hormone levels. Prospective randomized placebo-controlled trials [20, 21] have demonstrated the efficacy of a low-dose COCP which is licensed in the USA and Australia among other countries for treatment of PMDD. There are also generic versions of this pill and newer pills with estradiol and estetrol rather than ethinylestradiol which may be better tolerated by PMS/PMDD sufferers, although comparative data are lacking.

4.4.2 Estrogen and Progestogen/Progesterone Therapy

Percutaneous hormone replacement therapy in the form of estradiol implants or the transdermal patch has been shown to suppress ovarian activity and improve PMS/PMDD symptoms [22, 23]. Suppression of ovulation usually requires the use of higher doses of estradiol than is used in post-menopausal HRT, for example, 100 mcg estradiol patch.

In non-hysterectomized women, estradiol should be given in combination with a progestogen. Cyclical progestogenic opposition (10–12 days per cycle) is required to protect against endometrial hyperplasia. However, progestogens commonly result in worsening of PMS/PMDD symptoms, and therefore careful consideration should be given to this element of HRT. Fewer side effects are generally seen with bioidentical progesterone (typically 200 mg for 12 days per 28 day cycle), the levonorgestrel intrauterine system, or vaginal administered progesterone pessaries and gels.

There is no evidence to support the use of synthetic progestogens and little evidence to support the use of natural progesterone alone in the management of PMS [24].

4.4.3 GnRH Analogues

Some women will not respond to the above measures, and at this stage referral to specialist services should be made if the patient has been managed in primary care thus far. Inadequate response to treatment may be due to incomplete cycle suppression. GnRH analogues may be considered the next-line treatment and can be used to completely suppress ovarian activity and are of proven efficacy in the treatment of severe PMS/PMDD [25]. If GnRH analogues are used for longer than 6 months, they must be used in combination with "add-back" estrogen and progestogen hormone therapy to avoid symptoms of estrogen deficiency and its detrimental effects on bone density and metabolism. Although the addition of add-back hormone therapy has not been shown to reduce the efficacy of GnRHa [26], in a small proportion of women, it may lead to recurrence of their cyclical symptoms, in which case continuous tibolone is an alternative option. For long-term GnRH use, yearly assessment of bone density should be undertaken.

The recent development of the new oral GnRH antagonists, e.g., relugolix, elagolix, and linzagolix which can be used with add-back hormone therapy, could provide another treatment option for women with severe PMS/PMDD. The indication for these drugs currently is for the treatment of moderate to severe symptoms associated with uterine fibroids. Research is required to assess the impact of these treatments on PMS/PMDD symptoms and to determine the optimal add-back hormone regimens which would be required to avoid adverse effects in this group of hormone-sensitive women.

4.4.4 Surgical Options

For women with severe PMS/PMDD hysterectomy and bilateral oophorectomy, which can usually be performed laparoscopically, will provide permanent cycle suppression and is the only known "cure" for this condition. For those with severe PMS/PMDD who have completed their families, it can be a life-changing procedure. It is not without its risks and should only be considered in women who have demonstrated a response to GnRH analogues and who are able to tolerate hormone therapy so that cycle-related symptoms are not merely replaced by menopause symptoms. Bilateral oophorectomy alone is not recommended as endometrial protection with progestogens/progesterone will still be required and women with PMS/PMDD are often intolerant to these hormones.

Following the procedure, adequate hormone therapy should be given in women to avoid the effects of estrogen deficiency on quality of life and long-term well-being. Estradiol can be administered via implant, orally or transdermally. In the author's experience, anecdotally, women do better with implants post-surgery rather than other forms of hormone therapy due to the adequate constant hormone levels. Consideration should also be given to testosterone replacement, especially if suffering from symptoms of distressing low libido. Studies thus far have shown a good response with high satisfaction rates following this procedure [27].

4.4.5 New Research

A phase IIb placebo-controlled double-blinded trial was recently completed using Sepranolone in women with confirmed PMDD. Sepranolone is a GABA receptor modulator which regulates the effects of allopregnanolone in the central nervous system. Although numerically the symptom reduction was greater for the Sepranolone group than for the placebo group, the difference between the groups was not statistically significant, mainly because there was such a strong placebo effect [28]. It is hoped that further research will be conducted in the future using this or similar interventions where a placebo run in phase may eliminate some of the placebo effect before the subjects are randomized.

5 Conclusion

Severe PMS/PMDD causes significant impairment to daily functioning and quality of life and is often poorly diagnosed and managed. It is encouraging that PMDD has been recognized by the WHO in the International Classification of Diseases as this may lead to improved training and research to manage this distressing condition. Although the underlying etiology is still not fully understood, a number of treatments with demonstrated efficacy do exist. Unfortunately, despite favorable data, in most countries there are few or no treatment options available with a license for the PMS/PMDD indication.

Lifestyle and complementary approaches play a role, but better data are required. Often a combination of psychological and hormonal treatments are required; hence, more collaboration between psychiatrists and gynecologists is required to fully understand the synergistic benefits of these approaches. Despite advances in treatment options, some women will still benefit greatly from surgical management, but it is vital that this is coupled with adequate hormone therapy.

Online Healthcare Professional and Patient Support and Information

https://pms.org.uk
https://iapmd.org
https://rcog.org.uk
https://helloclue.com/
https://flo.health/

References

1. Magos AL, Studd JWW. The premenstrual syndrome. In: Studd J, editor. Progress in obstetrics and gynaecology, vol. 4. London: Churchill Livingstone; 1984. p. 334–50.
2. Panay N. Management of premenstrual syndrome. J Fam Plan Reprod Health Care. 2009;35:187–94.
3. American Psychiatric Association, editor. Diagnostic and statistical manual of mental disorders-DSM-IV. 4th ed. Washington, DC: American Psychiatric Association; 1994.
4. O'Brien PMS, Bäckström T, Brown C, et al. Towards a consensus on diagnostic criteria, measurement and trial design of the premenstrual disorders: the ISPMD Montreal consensus. Arch Womens Ment Health. 2011;14:13–21.
5. Nevatte T, O'Brien PM, Bäckström T, et al. Consensus Group of the International Society for Premenstrual Disorders. ISPMD consensus on the management of premenstrual disorders. Arch Womens Ment Health. 2013;16:279–91.
6. Green LJ, O'Brien PMS, Panay N, Craig M, on behalf of the Royal College of Obstetricians and Gynaecologists. Management of premenstrual syndrome. BJOG. 2017;124:e73–e105.
7. Goswami N, Upadhyay K, Briggs P, Osborn E, Panay N. Premenstrual disorders including premenstrual syndrome and premenstrual dysphoric disorder. Obstet Gynecol. 2023;25:38–46.
8. Rubinow DR, Hoban MC, Grover GN, Galloway DS, Roy-Byrne P, Andersen R, Merriam GR. Changes in plasma hormones across the menstrual cycle in patients with menstrually related mood disorder and in control subjects. Am J Obstet Gynecol. 1988;158:5–11.
9. Huo L, Straub RE, Roca C, Schmidt PJ, Shi K, Vakkalanka R, et al. Risk for premenstrual dysphoric disorder is associated with genetic variation in ESR1, the estrogen receptor alpha gene. Biol Psychiatry. 2007;62:925–33.
10. Dubey N, Hoffman JF, Schuebel K, Yuan Q, Martinez PE, Nieman LK, et al. The ESC/E (Z) complex, an effector of response to ovarian steroids, manifests an intrinsic difference in cells from women with premenstrual dysphoric disorder. Mol Psychiatry. 2017;22:1172–84.
11. Inoue Y, Terao T, Iwata N, Okamoto K, Kojima H, Okamoto T, et al. Fluctuating serotonergic function in premenstrual dysphoric disorder and premenstrual syndrome: findings from neuro-endocrine challenge tests. Psychopharmacology. 2007;190:213–9.
12. Rapkin AJ, Morgan M, Goldman L, et al. Progesterone metabolite allopregnanolone in women with premenstrual syndrome. Obstet Gynecol. 1997;90:709–14.
13. Studd J, Panay N. Hormones and depression in women. Climacteric. 2004;7(4):338–46.
14. Prior JC, Vigna Y, Sciarretta D, Alojado N, Schulzer M. Conditioning exercise decreases premenstrual symptoms: a prospective, controlled 6-month trial. Fertil Steril. 1987;47:402–8.
15. Hunter MS, Ussher JM, Browne SJ, Cariss M, Jelley R, Katz M. A randomized comparison of psychological (cognitive behaviour therapy), medical (fluoxetine) and combined treatment for women with premenstrual dysphoric disorder. J Psychosom Obstet Gynaecol. 2002;23:193–9.

16. Csupor D, Lantos T, Hegyi P, et al. Vitex agnus-castus in premenstrual syndrome: a meta-analysis of double-blind randomised controlled trials. Complement Ther Med. 2019;47:102190.
17. Brown J, O'Brien PM, Marjoribanks J, Wyatt K. Selective serotonin reuptake inhibitors for premenstrual syndrome. Cochrane Database Syst Rev. 2009;2:CD001396.
18. Cohen LS, Soares CN, Lyster AB, Cassano P, Brandes M, Leblanc G. Efficacy and tolerability of premenstrual use of venlafaxine (flexible dose) in the treatment of premenstrual dysphoric disorder. J Clin Psychopharmacol. 2004;24:540–3.
19. Freeman EW, Kroll R, Rapkin A, Pearlstein T, Brown C, Parsey K, PMS/PMDD Research Group, et al. Evaluation of a unique oral contraceptive in the treatment of premenstrual dysphoric disorder. J Womens Health Gend Based Med. 2001;10:561–9.
20. Pearlstein TB, Bachmann GA, Zacur HA, Yonkers KA. Treatment of premenstrual dysphoric disorder with a new drospirenone-containing oral contraceptive formulation. Contraception. 2005;72:414–21.
21. Yonkers KA, Brown C, Pearlstein TB, Foegh M, Sampson-Landers C, Rapkin A. Efficacy of a new low-dose oral contraceptive with drospirenone in premenstrual dysphoric disorder. Obstet Gynaecol. 2005;106:492–501.
22. Magos AL, Brincat M, Studd JWW. Treatment of the pre-menstrual syndrome by subcutaneous estradiol implants and cyclical oral norethisterone: placebo controlled study. Br Med J. 1986;292:1629–33.
23. Watson NR, Studd JW, Savvas M, Garnett T, Baber RJ. Treatment of severe premenstrual syndrome with estradiol patches and cyclical oral norethisterone. Lancet. 1989;ii:730–2.
24. Ford O, Lethaby A, Roberts H, Mol BW. Progesterone for premenstrual syndrome. Cochrane Database Syst Rev. 2009;2:CD003415.
25. Wyatt K, Dimmock P, Ismail K, Jones P, O'Brien P. The effectiveness of GnRHa with and without 'add-back' therapy in treating premenstrual syndrome: a meta-analysis. Br J Obstet Gynaecol. 2004;111(6):585–93.
26. Leather AT, Studd JW, Watson NR, Holland EF. The treatment of severe premenstrual syndrome with goserelin with and without 'add-back' estrogen therapy: a placebo-controlled study. Gynecol Endocrinol. 1999;13(1):48–55.
27. Cronje WH, Vashisht A, Studd JW. Hysterectomy and bilateral oophorectomy for severe premenstrual syndrome. Hum Reprod. 2004;19(9):2152–5.
28. Bäckström T, Ekberg K, Hirschberg AL, Bixo M, Epperson CN, Briggs P, Panay N, O'Brien S. A randomized, double-blind study on efficacy and safety of sepranolone in premenstrual dysphoric disorder. Psychoneuroendocrinology. 2021;133:105426.

Endometriosis and Adenomyosis

Silvia Vannuccini, Batuhan Aslan, and Felice Petraglia

1 Introduction

Adenomyosis and endometriosis are two different diseases, whose historical, pathological, and clinical association cannot be denied. While in the nineteenth century, French pathologists observed the first macroscopic findings of endometriosis in postmortem series [1], in 1860 an Austrian pathologist Karl von Rokitansky stated that endometrium-like stroma and glands may be found unexpectedly in ectopic locations [1]. Finally, in the twentieth century, Thomas Cullen coined the term "diffuse adenomyoma," and Sampson coined the term endometriosis [1], and the two conditions were recognized as separate pathological entities [2]. Both diseases are characterized by the presence of endometrial stroma and gland-like tissue in ectopic foci: adenomyosis, in the case of myometrial location, endometriosis when the ectopic endometrium is outside the uterus.

S. Vannuccini · F. Petraglia (✉)
Department of Experimental, Clinical and Biomedical Sciences "Mario Serio",
University of Florence, Florence, Italy

Obstetrics and Gynecology, Careggi University Hospital, Florence, Italy
e-mail: silvia.vannuccini@unifi.it; felice.petraglia@unifi.it

B. Aslan
Department of Obstetrics and Gynecology, Ankara University School of Medicine,
Ankara, Turkey

A. R. Genazzani et al. (eds.), *Menstrual Bleeding and Pain Disorders from Adolescence to Menopause*, ISGE Series,
https://doi.org/10.1007/978-3-031-55300-4_9

2 Pathogenesis of Adenomyosis

Adenomyosis is histologically defined as the presence of endometrial glands and stroma deep within the myometrium, and it is characterized by surrounding myometrial hypertrophy, hyperplasia, and fibrosis [3]. Lesions may be focal when localized in a myometrial area, while lesions distributed throughout the myometrium are defined as diffuse [4], but also a specific entity known as cystic adenomyoma is described [5].

Complex pathogenic mechanisms such as sex steroid hormone dysfunction, inflammation, abnormal immune response, cell migration, invasion and proliferation, fibrosis, and neuroangiogenesis are involved in the development of adenomyosis [6].

The origin of adenomyosis considers different theories. The invagination hypothesis primarily relies on the tissue injury and repair (TIAR) mechanism [7]. The TIAR phenomenon assumes the migration of the endometrium through an altered, injured, or abnormal junctional zone (JZ), at the endometrial-myometrial interface (EMI), invading into the myometrium, upon myocyte and fibroblast damage. This mechanism seems to be caused by sustained trauma and myometrial strain, as a result of occurring myometrial hyperperistalsis. The consequent microtrauma causes a vicious circle (auto-traumatization) with increased inflammation and local estrogen production; thus, uterine hyperperistalsis is further stimulated through the activation of estrogen receptors (ERs) and oxytocin receptor system [7]. Chronic hypercontractility and autotraumatization contribute to the development of adenomyosis.

The metaplasia theory includes differentiation of embryonic pluripotent Müllerian cells or stem cells, which causes the development of *de novo* adenomyotic foci within the myometrium [6]. This theory may be especially acceptable in explaining the adenomyosis observed in rudimentary uterine structures in case of Mayer-Rokitansky-Küster-Hauser syndrome [4].

Another hypothesis suggests that ectopic endometrial cells penetrating the uterine wall and forming a uterine adenomyotic nodule may extend posteriorly toward the outer wall of the rectum predisposing to the development of deep infiltrating endometriosis (DIE) nodules [4]. More likely is the opposite way round, which assumes the migration of ectopic cells from DIE nodules into the myometrium ("outside-to-inside theory") [8], as supported by the frequent association of posterior focal adenomyosis of the outer myometrium (FOAM) and DIE in the posterior compartment [9, 10]. On this background, it has been suggested that diffuse adenomyosis originates from the subendometrial migration of eutopic endometrium ("inside-to-inside theory"), whereas focal adenomyosis originates from the invasion of the myometrium by endometriotic cells [11].

3   Pathogenesis of Endometriosis

Endometriosis is an estrogen-dependent, chronic, and inflammatory disease characterized by the ectopic presence of endometrial stroma and glands in extrauterine tissues [12]. Mainly, the ovaries, peritoneum, uterosacral ligaments, rectovaginal septum, rectum, and bladder are affected [13]. According to their main location, there are three phenotypes: ovarian (OMA), peritoneal (superficial) (SUP), and DIE.

The theories explaining the pathophysiology of endometriosis include retrograde menstruation and implantation, coelomic metaplasia, direct transplantation, and vascular/lymphatic spread. Although none of these possible mechanisms is sufficient to explain the pathogenesis of endometriosis alone, nowadays the most accepted is the retrograde menstruation theory proposed by Sampson in 1927 [14]. Accordingly, endometrial tissue shed during menstruation is transported to the peritoneal space via the fallopian tubes and steroid-sensitive endometrial cell implant on the pelvic organs and causes an inflammatory response. As a result angiogenesis, adhesion, fibrosis and scar formation, neuronal infiltration, and anatomical distortion occur, resulting in pain and infertility [15]. In addition, the inability to clean the implants from the peritoneal surface due to the immune system disorder is thought to have a role in the development of the disease. The common pelvic localizations and the fact that endometriosis is frequent in adolescents with obstructive genital anomalies than in those without support the retrograde menstruation theory [16].

According to the coelomic metaplasia theory, endometriosis develops with metaplastic changes from mesothelial cells of coelomic epithelial origin such as the pleura, pericardium, peritoneum, and omentum [17–19]. The occurrence of endometriosis in patients with Mayer-Rokitansky-Küster-Hauser syndrome with complete uterine agenesis [24] and in men [25] supports this theory [20]. Although coelomic metaplasia may be an explanation for peritoneal and pleural endometriosis, it does not account for intestinal or pulmonary parenchymal involvement. The embryonic Müllerian remnant, or Mullerianosis theory, claims that cells from embryological Müllerian duct migration retain the capacity to develop into endometriotic lesions in response to the action of estrogen, which begins at puberty [21].

Any of the theories outlined above cannot fully explain endometriosis. Therefore, different concepts have been combined to understand the disease's pathogenesis and the different types of endometriosis. For instance, the composite theory combines the theories of implantation, lymphatic spread, and direct spread of endometriosis. While ovarian and deep endometriosis lesions can be explained by metaplasia, peritoneal lesions may occur due to implantation.

4 Pathogenetic Factors of Endometriosis and Adenomyosis

4.1 The Role of Gonadal Sex Steroid Hormones

Sex steroid hormones, estrogen and progesterone, play a crucial role in the origin and development of adenomyosis and endometriosis [8, 22] (Fig. 1).

The hyperestrogenism with normal peripheral serum estradiol levels is related to altered estrogen receptor ER-α function and to a local estrogen production, both in endometriosis and adenomyosis, probably due to the activation of TIAR mechanisms induced by microtrauma at the basal endometrial layer level [23]. Basal endometrial fragments into the peritoneal cavity can induce mechanisms of chronic inflammation and activate local estrogen production, cell proliferation, and infiltrative growth resulting in endometriosis [23]. Moreover, the effect of 17β-hydroxysteroid dehydrogenase type 2 (17β-HSD2) in the eutopic endometrium

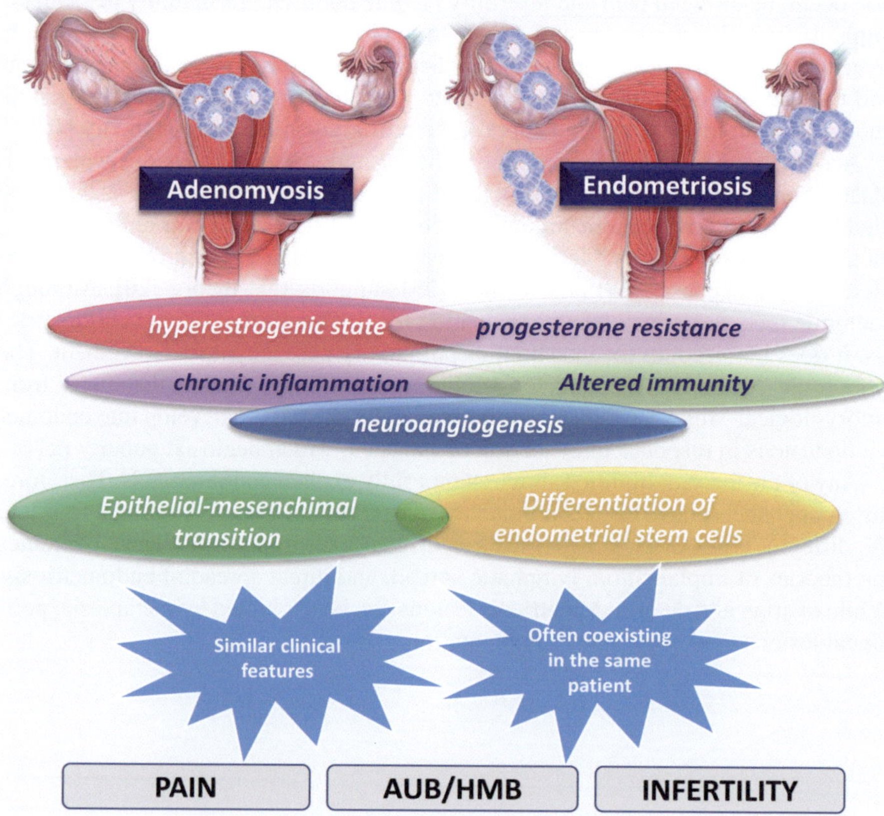

Fig. 1 Common pathogenetic mechanisms and clinical presentation of endometriosis and adenomyosis

in both endometriosis and adenomyosis results in decreased local estrogen metabolism due to its altered regulation [8, 23].

4.2   The Role of Immune Factors

An abnormal immune response is common in women with adenomyosis or endometriosis (Fig. 1). Different immune-related markers vary at the systemic level and locally in the eutopic and ectopic endometrium. T cell populations and macrophages are increased in the eutopic endometrium of women with adenomyosis or endometriosis, supporting the concept that both innate and adaptive immunities play a role in the development of the two diseases [8]. Epithelial-to-mesenchymal transition (EMT) and sustained infiltration by inflammatory macrophages can lead to fibrosis, while inflammatory mediators may interfere with other physiological functions, such as embryo implantation [4]. Transcriptomic analysis of the endometrium of women with endometriosis revealed altered steroid hormone signaling and upregulation of pathways, including lymphocyte activation, antigen presentation, cytokine induction, and inflammation. In women with endometriosis, immune and inflammation endometrial genes reveal alterations in endometrial stromal fibroblast cellular apoptosis and progesterone-induced decidualization [24].

4.3   The Role of Inflammation and Neurogenesis

A relevant role of inflammatory processes in adenomyosis and endometriosis development is well established [25] (Fig. 1). Ectopic endometrial tissues induce an inflammatory peritoneal environment that adversely affects uterine steroid response. Interleukin (IL)-1β, IL-6, IL-8, corticotropin-releasing hormone, urocortin, synaptophysin, and microtubule-associated protein 2 are highly expressed in adenomyotic nodules compared to the eutopic endometrium [8]. Moreover, cyclooxygenase 2 (COX-2) is overexpressed in the eutopic and ectopic endometrium of adenomyosis and appears to play a critical role in the pathogenesis of the disease [8]. Increased concentrations of various inflammatory cytokines (e.g., IL-6, IL-8, and tumor necrosis factor alpha (TNF-a)), growth factors (e.g., vascular endothelial growth factor (VEGF)), and pain mediators (mainly prostaglandin E2 (PGE2)) are observed in endometriosis compared to normal peritoneal fluid [26]. It has been suggested that the local and systemic hyperinflammatory environment and the abnormal hormonal environment associated with endometriosis promote also the development of adenomyosis [27]. Moreover, environmental toxicants that act as endocrine-disrupting chemicals can affect the pathogenesis of both diseases [27].

Histamine, serotonin, bradykinin, PGs, leukotriene, ILs, acetylcholine, and nerve growth factor (NGF) are potent allogenic factors responsible for the functional and structural changes of nociceptors. They cause an increase in nerve fibers' excitability (peripheral sensitization) and explain pain symptoms both in adenomyosis and endometriosis [8, 28]. Increased expression of NGFs, synaptophysin, and NF proteins may explain the higher perception of uterine pain in adenomyosis [29]. Increased expression of nerve growth factor, increased density of nerve fibers, angiogenesis, and changes in the innervation of the uterus may also contribute [30].

5 Epidemiology and Risk Factors of Endometriosis and Adenomyosis

The prevalence and risk factors of adenomyosis are currently uncertain [31–33]. The disease has historically been identified as a pathological entity from histological reports after hysterectomy. Recent diagnostic advances have enabled the detection of adenomyosis with less invasive methods, such as transvaginal ultrasound (TVUS) and magnetic resonance (MRI). The prevalence of the disease in adolescence and young women is still a matter of debate. According to TVUS, the overall prevalence of adenomyosis is 20.9% [31]. The frequency increases with age, reaching a peak of 32% in women aged 40–49 [31]. However, it has been reported that adenomyosis is detected in approximately 45% of young women complaining of chronic pelvic pain [32]. The most common risk factors include being over 40 years of age, multiparity, prior delivery, or uterine surgery [6]. Adenomyosis is reported to be identified between 20% and 25% of women undergoing assisted reproductive technologies (ART), whereas this rate varies widely (20–60%) in those with a history of endometriosis [6]. A higher prevalence of adenomyosis also has been reported in women treated with tamoxifen for breast cancer [33]. The neoplastic potential in adenomyosis has not yet been established [34].

Endometriosis is a complex inflammatory syndrome that affects women throughout the reproductive age from adolescence. Despite the advancements in imaging technologies and basic science, a reliable, non-invasive gold standard method for diagnosis of endometriosis has not been found yet. Therefore, it varies between 2% and 10% in the general female population, up to 50% of infertile women [35, 36]. The mean time of diagnosis is between 25 and 35 years, and a wide range of patients with chronic pelvic pain are diagnosed in adolescence [37–39]. Although it is less common in adolescents, it is detected in 62% of women younger than 20 with chronic pelvic pain, dysmenorrhea, or dyspareunia [40]. The prevalence varies between 2% and 11% in asymptomatic women, 5% and 50% in infertile women, and 5% and 21% in women hospitalized for pelvic pain, even though figures are not fully representative [41]. The prevalence of endometriosis in adolescents with chronic pelvic pain who does not respond to medical therapy ranges from 49% to 75% [41].

Although the exact cause is unknown, it is seen more in Asians than in white women and less in black ethnicity [42]. The frequency of endometriosis is inversely related to body mass index (BMI) and is more common in thin women [42]. Early menarche, short menstrual cycle, and heavy menstrual bleeding (HMB) increase the risk of endometriosis [43, 44]. Pregnancy, multiparity, and prolonged lactation reduce the risk of endometriosis [45]. While alcohol and caffeine consumption is associated with an increased risk of endometriosis, smoking is associated with a decreased risk [42, 46, 47]. Nickel allergy appears to be a risk factor for endometriosis [48]. It is generally associated with a minimal and insignificantly increased risk of cancer, based on a systematic review and meta-analysis of 49 recently published cohort or case-control studies [49].

6   Clinical Presentation of Endometriosis and Adenomyosis

The high rate of co-occurrence of diseases makes it difficult to evaluate them separately (Fig. 1). It was reported that 42.3% of women diagnosed with endometriosis also had adenomyosis [50, 51].

6.1   Pain

One of the main symptoms of adenomyosis and endometriosis is pelvic pain. Dysmenorrhea and dyspareunia are explained by inflammatory factors (IL-1β and corticotropin-releasing hormone) and increased COX and PGs levels [29, 52]. Pain in endometriosis results also from compression and/or infiltration of adjacent organs and nerves [30]. In particular, endometriosis of bowel and bladder may be associated with dyschezia and dysuria. Besides, endometriosis is also associated to a central pain syndrome (fibromyalgia, migraine, back pain).

6.2   Abnormal Uterine Bleeding (AUB)

HMB and premenstrual and postmenstrual spotting are typical symptoms of adenomyosis, for both endometrial and myometrial causes. The eutopic endometrium in adenomyosis presents an abnormal hormonal background with a disturbed response to progesterone, contributing to HMB [53]. The activation of coagulation and fibrinolysis system has been found to be activated at the time of menstruation in women with   adenomyosis,   contributing   to   HMB   via   the   formation   of   local microhemorrhage and microthrombi [53]. Increased angiogenesis and fragile vascular structure also contribute to bleeding [54]. In these patients, iron deficiency anemia is noteworthy [55]. Endometriosis patients present with AUB when adenomyosis is associated.

6.3 Infertility

Patients with adenomyosis have lower clinical pregnancy rates, lower live birth rates, higher miscarriage rates, and a higher chance of adverse obstetric outcomes [56]. Although the guidelines do not recommend a specific treatment protocol for adenomyosis, medical and surgical approaches have the effect of increasing pregnancy and live birth rates [56]. In endometriosis, anatomical changes, a decreased ovarian reserve, and a local inflammatory response of peritoneal ectopic endometrial foci contribute to the observed infertility [57]. Endometriosis is diagnosed in 35–40% of women with infertility [58]. Especially in view of the increasing age of women wishing to conceive, ART-priority approaches are recommended increasingly in endometriosis patients [58]. However, in a number of cases, surgery may be preferable to increase the chances of conceiving naturally, provided there is time (age and ovarian reserve) to conceive spontaneously [58]. Patient-based assessment is the best approach in endometriosis women with desire of pregnancy.

6.4 Systemic Comorbidities

There is a relationship between endometriosis and gastrointestinal, inflammatory, metabolic, and immunological diseases [44]. Irritable bowel syndrome, celiac, lactose intolerance, rheumatoid arthritis, psoriasis, and migraine are the main associated diseases [44, 59]. Endometriosis was associated with a higher risk of ovarian and thyroid cancer, although the causal link needs to be further assessed [49]. Regarding adenomyosis, so far there is no evidence of the association with other diseases, except for IDA resulting from HMB, and the well-known coexistence with endometriosis and other uterine disorders, such as uterine fibroids.

7 Diagnosis

The precise diagnosis of adenomyosis is based on the presence of ectopic endometrial tissue in the myometrium by pathological analysis [60]. In the last 15 years, the diagnosis of adenomyosis has been accessible by TVUS and MRI, even though some limitations in imaging accuracy and standardization still remain [3]. Ultrasound criteria for diagnosing adenomyosis using Morphological Uterus Sonographic

Assessment (MUSA) are well defined: asymmetrical thickening of the uterine walls, intramyometrial cysts or hyperechoic islands (or both), fan-shaped shadowing of the myometrium, myometrial echogenic subendometrial lines, and buds, translesional vascularity, and irregular or interrupted junctional zone (JZ) [61]. Diagnosis is made by the presence of at least one of these criteria: 84% and 64% specificity and sensitivity, respectively, are reported [62]. Pelvic MRI is a more expensive, with reproducible examination; specificity and sensitivity of MRI are thought to be 77.5% and 92.5%, respectively [60].

The diagnosis of endometriosis was previously made by histopathological demonstration of ectopically located endometrial stroma and gland tissue, but TVUS and MRI are becoming alternative reliable methods for diagnosing the disease. Pain in the form of dysmenorrhea, dyspareunia, chronic pelvic pain, or multiple accompanying symptoms is common in patients with endometriosis [63, 64]. Depending on the extent of endometriosis, additional painful symptoms may be observed in the urinary and gastrointestinal regions. Physical examination of the pelvis and abdomen is necessary to facilitate diagnosis and optimize treatment decisions [65]: palpable tender nodules or a thickened area containing any of several pelvic regions (torus uterinus, uterosacral ligament(s), upper third of posterior vaginal wall, pouch of Douglas), adnexal mass, and rigid retroverted uterus [65–68]. TVUS and MRI are suitable for diagnosing the two phenotypes of endometriosis (ovarian and DIE) and for the concurrent evaluation of adenomyosis [66, 67]. In addition, sigmoid, ileocecal, and urinary tract lesions may be detected by complementary radiological techniques [68]. The TVUS criteria are determined by the International Analysis of Deep Endometriosis (IDEA) group recommending a systematic approach to evaluating pelvic sonography in patients with suspected endometriosis, showing a good accuracy for OMA (93% sensitivity and 96% specificity) and DIE (79% sensitivity and 94% specificity) [68]. However, SUP lesions are hardly identified by imaging [68]. MRI is the second-line technique allowing also the detection of extrapelvic endometriosis [69]. When both techniques were applied in the same patients, the diagnostic performances of TVUS (85% sensitivity and 96% specificity) and MRI (85% sensitivity and 95% specificity) were similar to detecting rectosigmoid DIE [70].

8 Management

Adenomyosis and endometriosis have a negative impact on women's quality of life due to pain, infertility, and AUB requiring a lifelong management plan through medical, surgical, or infertility treatment. The choice depends on the symptoms, woman's age, desire of pregnancy, and clinical history. The surgical treatment option for adenomyosis has not been generally accepted, while surgery is considered an appropriate treatment option for endometriosis in managing pain and infertility, even if it should be minimally invasive.

Although surgery remains an important management strategy for endometriosis, it should not be forgotten that it does not treat the underlying cause of the disease and is associated with a high recurrence rate [71]. Especially in cases of DIE, significant complications of surgery are noteworthy (e.g., postoperative infection, rectovaginal fistula, neurogenic bladder, and bowel dysfunction). In addition, the potential adverse effect of OMA on ovarian reserve after laparoscopic cystectomy requires appropriate management in women who desire subsequent pregnancy [72]. Medical treatment is a good alternative to surgery (progestins, GnRH analogs, oral GnRH antagonists) and may help in planning a fertility-sparing or surgical management. Postoperative medical treatment option is suggested to prevent the disease recurrence after the operation and prevent pain (unless the patient has no desire of pregnancy) [72]. For adenomyosis, hormonal treatment is the most suggested (levonorgestrel-releasing intrauterine system, progestins, GnRH analogs, oral GnRH antagonists), and conservative surgical/radiological options (endometrial ablation, hysteroscopic endometrial resection of adenomyosis, high-intensity focused ultrasonography, and uterine artery embolization) remain an alternative option [73]. Current medical treatments for endometriosis and adenomyosis include also non-hormonal treatments such as pain relievers and NSAIDs. Medical treatment should be the first choice in the treatment of pain and inflammation due to endometriosis in patients who do not want to become pregnant.

9 Conclusion

Adenomyosis and endometriosis are diseases with similar pathogenetic processes and are frequently observed together. The heterogeneous clinical presentation observed in both diseases complicates the diagnosis and follow-up of patients and often prolongs the time from symptom onset to diagnosis. TVUS and MRI are useful for the diagnosis of both diseases, due to the advancements in technologies and the increased awareness among clinicians. Endometriosis is also associated with systemic comorbidities, while adenomyosis is more likely associated with IDA, resulting from HMB. Psychological problems are common with impairment in social and work life, loss of productivity, and economic damage. An holistic approach and a tailored management is advisable to take care of women affected by endometriosis and adenomyosis.

References

1. Nezhat C, Nezhat F, Nezhat C. Endometriosis: ancient disease, ancient treatments. Fertil Steril. 2012;98(6):S1–S62.
2. Benagiano G, Brosens I. Adenomyosis and endometriosis have a common origin. J Obstet Gynecol India. 2011;61(2):146–52.

3. Loring M, Chen TY, Isaacson KB. A systematic review of adenomyosis: it is time to reassess what we thought we knew about the disease. J Minim Invasive Gynecol. 2021;28(3):644–55.

4. Stratopoulou CA, Donnez J, Dolmans M-M. Origin and pathogenic mechanisms of uterine adenomyosis: what is known so far. Reprod Sci. 2021;28(8):2087–97.

5. Brosens I, Gordts S, Habiba M, Benagiano G. Uterine cystic adenomyosis: a disease of younger women. J Pediatr Adolesc Gynecol. 2015;28(6):420–6.

6. Vannuccini S, Petraglia F. Recent advances in understanding and managing adenomyosis [version 1; peer review: 2 approved]. F1000Res. 2019;8(283):283.

7. Leyendecker G, Wildt L. A new concept of endometriosis and adenomyosis: tissue injury and repair (TIAR). Horm Mol Biol Clin Invest. 2011;5(2):125–42.

8. Vannuccini S, Tosti C, Carmona F, Huang SJ, Chapron C, Guo S-W, et al. Pathogenesis of adenomyosis: an update on molecular mechanisms. Reprod Biomed Online. 2017;35(5):592–601.

9. Chapron C, Tosti C, Marcellin L, Bourdon M, Lafay-Pillet M-C, Millischer A-E, et al. Relationship between the magnetic resonance imaging appearance of adenomyosis and endometriosis phenotypes. Hum Reprod. 2017;32(7):1393–401.

10. Donnez J, Dolmans M-M, Fellah L. What if deep endometriotic nodules and uterine adenomyosis were actually two forms of the same disease? Fertil Steril. 2019;111(3):454–6.

11. Bourdon M, Santulli P, Jeljeli M, Vannuccini S, Marcellin L, Doridot L, et al. Immunological changes associated with adenomyosis: a systematic review. Hum Reprod Update. 2021;27(1):108–29.

12. Bulun SE, Yilmaz BD, Sison C, Miyazaki K, Bernardi L, Liu S, et al. Endometriosis. Endocr Rev. 2019;40(4):1048–79.

13. Macer ML, Taylor HS. Endometriosis and infertility: a review of the pathogenesis and treatment of endometriosis-associated infertility. Obstet Gynecol Clin. 2012;39(4):535–49.

14. Sampson JA. Peritoneal endometriosis due to menstrual dissemination of endometrial tissue into the peritoneal cavity. Am J Obstet Gynecol. 1927;14:422–69.

15. Burney RO, Giudice LC. Pathogenesis and pathophysiology of endometriosis. Fertil Steril. 2012;98(3):511–9.

16. Yang Y, Wang Y, Yang J, Wang S, Lang J. Adolescent endometriosis in China: a retrospective analysis of 63 cases. J Pediatr Adolesc Gynecol. 2012;25(5):295–9.

17. Meyer R. Zur Frage der heterotopen Epithelwucherung, insbesondere des Peritonealepithels und in den Ovarien. Virchows Arch Pathol Anat Physiol Klin Med. 1924;250(3):595–610.

18. Ferguson BR, Bennington JL, Haber SL. Histochemistry of mucosubstances and histology of mixed müllerian pelvic lymph node glandular inclusions: evidence for histogenesis by müllerian metaplasia of coelomic epithelium. Obstet Gynecol. 1969;33(5):617–25.

19. Ganshina I. Serous cavities of coelomic origin as possible organs of the immune system. Part 1. Biol Bull Rev. 2016;6(6):497–504.

20. Mok-Lin EY, Wolfberg A, Hollinquist H, Laufer MR. Endometriosis in a patient with Mayer-Rokitansky-Küster-Hauser syndrome and complete uterine agenesis: evidence to support the theory of coelomic metaplasia. J Pediatr Adolesc Gynecol. 2010;23(1):e35–e7.

21. Batt RE, Smith RA, Buck Louis GM, Martin DC, Chapron C, Koninckx PR, et al. Müllerianosis. Histol Histopathol. 2007;22(10):1161–6.

22. Clemenza S, Capezzuoli T, Eren E, Garcia Garcia JM, Vannuccini S, Petraglia F. Progesterone receptor ligands for the treatment of endometriosis. Minerva Obstet Gynecol. 2022;75(3):288–97.

23. Laganà AS, Garzon S, Götte M, Viganò P, Franchi M, Ghezzi F, et al. The pathogenesis of endometriosis: molecular and cell biology insights. Int J Mol Sci. 2019;20(22):5615.

24. Vallvé-Juanico J, Houshdaran S, Giudice LC. The endometrial immune environment of women with endometriosis. Hum Reprod Update. 2019;25(5):564–91.

25. Reis FM, Petraglia F, Taylor RN. Endometriosis: hormone regulation and clinical consequences of chemotaxis and apoptosis. Hum Reprod Update. 2013;19(4):406–18.

26. Gruber TM, Mechsner S. Pathogenesis of endometriosis: the origin of pain and subfertility. Cell. 2021;10(6):1381.

27. Stephens VR, Rumph JT, Ameli S, Bruner-Tran KL, Osteen KG. The potential relationship between environmental endocrine disruptor exposure and the development of endometriosis and adenomyosis. Front Physiol. 2021;12:807685.
28. Tosti C, Pinzauti S, Santulli P, Chapron C, Petraglia F. Pathogenetic mechanisms of deep infiltrating endometriosis. Reprod Sci. 2015;22(9):1053–9.
29. Zhai J, Vannuccini S, Petraglia F, Giudice LC. Adenomyosis: mechanisms and pathogenesis. Semin Reprod Med. 2020;38(2–03):129–43.
30. Sachedina A, Todd N. Dysmenorrhea, endometriosis and chronic pelvic pain in adolescents. J Clin Res Pediatr Endocrinol. 2020;12(Suppl 1):7–17.
31. Naftalin J, Hoo W, Pateman K, Mavrelos D, Holland T, Jurkovic D. How common is adenomyosis? A prospective study of prevalence using transvaginal ultrasound in a gynaecology clinic. Hum Reprod. 2012;27(12):3432–9.
32. Zannoni L, Del Forno S, Raimondo D, Arena A, Giaquinto I, Paradisi R, et al. Adenomyosis and endometriosis in adolescents and young women with pelvic pain: prevalence and risk factors. Minerva Pediatr. 2020;
33. Kossaï M, Penault-Llorca F. Role of hormones in common benign uterine lesions: endometrial polyps, leiomyomas, and adenomyosis. In: Hormonal Pathology of the Uterus. Springer; 2020. p. 37–58.
34. Szubert M, Kozirog E, Wilczynski J. Adenomyosis as a risk factor for myometrial or endometrial neoplasms-review. Int J Environ Res Public Health. 2022;19(4):2294.
35. Fritz MA, Speroff L. Clinical gynecologic endocrinology and infertility. Lippincott Williams & Wilkins; 2012.
36. Meuleman C, Vandenabeele B, Fieuws S, Spiessens C, Timmerman D, D'Hooghe T. High prevalence of endometriosis in infertile women with normal ovulation and normospermic partners. Fertil Steril. 2009;92(1):68–74.
37. Kuohung W, Jones GL, Vitonis AF, Cramer DW, Kennedy SH, Thomas D, et al. Characteristics of patients with endometriosis in the United States and the United Kingdom. Fertil Steril. 2002;78(4):767–72.
38. Brosens I, Gordts S, Benagiano G. Endometriosis in adolescents is a hidden, progressive and severe disease that deserves attention, not just compassion. Hum Reprod. 2013;28(8):2026–31.
39. Shah DK, Missmer SA. Scientific investigation of endometriosis among adolescents. J Pediatr Adolesc Gynecol. 2011;24(5):S18–S9.
40. Janssen E, Rijkers A, Hoppenbrouwers K, Meuleman C, d'Hooghe T. Prevalence of endometriosis diagnosed by laparoscopy in adolescents with dysmenorrhea or chronic pelvic pain: a systematic review. Hum Reprod Update. 2013;19(5):570–82.
41. Zondervan KT, Becker CM, Missmer SA. Endometriosis. N Engl J Med. 2020;382(13):1244–56.
42. Missmer SA, Hankinson SE, Spiegelman D, Barbieri RL, Marshall LM, Hunter DJ. Incidence of laparoscopically confirmed endometriosis by demographic, anthropometric, and lifestyle factors. Am J Epidemiol. 2004;160(8):784–96.
43. Shafrir AL, Farland L, Shah D, Harris H, Kvaskoff M, Zondervan K, et al. Risk for and consequences of endometriosis: a critical epidemiologic review. Best Pract Res Clin Obstet Gynaecol. 2018;51:1–15.
44. Parazzini F, Esposito G, Tozzi L, Noli S, Bianchi S. Epidemiology of endometriosis and its comorbidities. Eur J Obstet Gynecol Reprod Biol. 2017;209:3–7.
45. Viganò P, Parazzini F, Somigliana E, Vercellini P. Endometriosis: epidemiology and aetiological factors. Best Pract Res Clin Obstet Gynaecol. 2004;18(2):177–200.
46. Zhou Y, Jorgensen EM, Gan Y, Taylor HS. Cigarette smoke increases progesterone receptor and homeobox A10 expression in human endometrium and endometrial cells: a potential role in the decreased prevalence of endometrial pathology in smokers. Biol Reprod. 2011;84(6):1242–7.
47. Hemmert R, Schliep KC, Willis S, Peterson CM, Louis GB, Allen-Brady K, et al. Modifiable life style factors and risk for incident endometriosis. Paediatr Perinat Epidemiol. 2019;33(1):19–25.

48. Yuk J-S, Shin JS, Shin J-Y, Oh E, Kim H, Park WI. Nickel allergy is a risk factor for endometriosis: an 11-year population-based nested case-control study. PLoS One. 2015;10(10):e0139388.

49. Kvaskoff M, Mahamat-Saleh Y, Farland LV, Shigesi N, Terry KL, Harris HR, et al. Endometriosis and cancer: a systematic review and meta-analysis. Hum Reprod Update. 2021;27(2):393–420.

50. Antero MF, O'Sullivan D, Mandavilli S, Mullins J. High prevalence of endometriosis in patients with histologically proven adenomyosis. Fertil Steril. 2017;107(3):e46.

51. Pinzauti S, Lazzeri L, Tosti C, Centini G, Orlandini C, Luisi S, et al. Transvaginal sonographic features of diffuse adenomyosis in 18–30-year-old nulligravid women without endometriosis: association with symptoms. Ultrasound Obstet Gynecol. 2015;46(6):730–6.

52. Machairiotis N, Vasilakaki S, Thomakos N. Inflammatory mediators and pain in endometriosis: a systematic review. Biomedicines. 2021;9(1):54.

53. Vannuccini S, Jain V, Critchley H, Petraglia F. From menarche to menopause, heavy menstrual bleeding is the underrated compass in reproductive health. Fertil Steril. 2022;118(4):625–36.

54. Harmsen MJ, Wong CF, Mijatovic V, Griffioen AW, Groenman F, Hehenkamp WJ, et al. Role of angiogenesis in adenomyosis-associated abnormal uterine bleeding and subfertility: a systematic review. Hum Reprod Update. 2019;25(5):647–71.

55. Petraglia F, Dolmans MM. Iron deficiency anemia: impact on women's reproductive health. Fertil Steril. 2022;118(4):605–6.

56. Moawad G, Kheil MH, Ayoubi JM, Klebanoff JS, Rahman S, Sharara FI. Adenomyosis and infertility. J Assist Reprod Genet. 2022;39(5):1027–31.

57. Broi MGD, Ferriani RA, Navarro PA. Ethiopathogenic mechanisms of endometriosis-related infertility. JBRA Assist Reprod. 2019;23(3):273–80.

58. Pirtea P, Vulliemoz N, de Ziegler D, Ayoubi JM. Infertility workup: identifying endometriosis. Fertil Steril. 2022;118:29.

59. Jenabi E, Khazaei S. Endometriosis and migraine headache risk: a meta-analysis. Women Health. 2020;60(8):939–45.

60. Bourdon M, Santulli P, Marcellin L, Maignien C, Maitrot-Mantelet L, Bordonne C, et al. Adenomyosis: an update regarding its diagnosis and clinical features. J Gynecol Obstet Hum Reprod. 2021;50(10):102228.

61. Van den Bosch T, Dueholm M, Leone F, Valentin L, Rasmussen C, Votino A, et al. Terms, definitions and measurements to describe sonographic features of myometrium and uterine masses: a consensus opinion from the Morphological Uterus Sonographic Assessment (MUSA) group. Ultrasound Obstet Gynecol. 2015;46(3):284–98.

62. Andres MP, Borrelli GM, Ribeiro J, Baracat EC, Abrão MS, Kho RM. Transvaginal ultrasound for the diagnosis of adenomyosis: systematic review and meta-analysis. J Minim Invasive Gynecol. 2018;25(2):257–64.

63. Sinaii N, Plumb K, Cotton L, Lambert A, Kennedy S, Zondervan K, et al. Differences in characteristics among 1,000 women with endometriosis based on extent of disease. Fertil Steril. 2008;89(3):538–45.

64. Chapron C, Lang J-H, Leng J-H, Zhou Y, Zhang X, Xue M, et al. Factors and regional differences associated with endometriosis: a multi-country, case–control study. Adv Ther. 2016;33(8):1385–407.

65. Bazot M, Lafont C, Rouzier R, Roseau G, Thomassin-Naggara I, Daraï E. Diagnostic accuracy of physical examination, transvaginal sonography, rectal endoscopic sonography, and magnetic resonance imaging to diagnose deep infiltrating endometriosis. Fertil Steril. 2009;92(6):1825–33.

66. Van den Bosch T, Van Schoubroeck D. Ultrasound diagnosis of endometriosis and adenomyosis: state of the art. Best Pract Res Clin Obstet Gynaecol. 2018;51:16–24.

67. Van den Bosch T, De Bruijn A, De Leeuw R, Dueholm M, Exacoustos C, Valentin L, et al. Sonographic classification and reporting system for diagnosing adenomyosis. Ultrasound Obstet Gynecol. 2019;53(5):576–82.

68. Nisenblat V, Bossuyt PM, Farquhar C, Johnson N, Hull ML. Imaging modalities for the non-invasive diagnosis of endometriosis. Cochrane Database Syst Rev. 2016;2:CD009591.

69. Foti PV, Farina R, Palmucci S, Vizzini IAA, Libertini N, Coronella M, et al. Endometriosis: clinical features, MR imaging findings and pathologic correlation. Insights Imaging. 2018;9(2):149–72.
70. Guerriero S, Saba L, Pascual M, Ajossa S, Rodriguez I, Mais V, et al. Transvaginal ultrasound vs magnetic resonance imaging for diagnosing deep infiltrating endometriosis: systematic review and meta-analysis. Ultrasound Obstet Gynecol. 2018;51(5):586–95.
71. Vercellini P, Crosignani P, Abbiati A, Somigliana E, Vigano P, Fedele L. The effect of surgery for symptomatic endometriosis: the other side of the story. Hum Reprod Update. 2009;15(2):177–88.
72. Chapron C, Marcellin L, Borghese B, Santulli P. Rethinking mechanisms, diagnosis and management of endometriosis. Nat Rev Endocrinol. 2019;15(11):666–82.
73. Dueholm M. Minimally invasive treatment of adenomyosis. Best Pract Res Clin Obstet Gynaecol. 2018;51:119–37.

Uterine Fibroids and Heavy Menstrual Bleeding

E. Casula, S. Macaluso, Andrea Giannini, S. Luisi, P. Mannella, Marta Caretto, Andrea R. Genazzani, and Tommaso Simoncini

1   Introduction

Uterine fibroids (also referred to as leiomyomas or myomas) are the most common pelvic neoplasm in females [1]. They are noncancerous monoclonal tumors arising from the smooth muscle cells and fibroblast of the myometrium. Incidence is difficult to determine since there are few longitudinal studies. They arise in reproductive-age females and, when symptomatic, typically present with abnormal uterine bleeding (AUB) and/or pelvic pain.

2   Fibroid Locations

Uterine fibroids are described according to their location in the uterus.

The International Federation of Gynecology and Obstetrics (FIGO) classification system [2] is stratified into nine basic categories that are arranged according to the acronym PALM-COEIN: polyp, adenomyosis, leiomyoma, malignancy and hyperplasia, coagulopathy, ovulatory disorders, endometrium, iatrogenic, and not classified. In general, the components of the PALM group are structural entities that are measurable visually, by use of imaging techniques, and/or by use of histopathology, while the COEIN group is related to entities that are not defined by imaging or

E. Casula · S. Macaluso · A. Giannini (✉) · S. Luisi · P. Mannella · M. Caretto ·
A. R. Genazzani · T. Simoncini
Department of Clinical and Experimental Medicine, Division of Obstetrics and Gynecology,
University of Pisa, Pisa, Italy
e-mail: andrea.giannini@unipi.it; tommso.simoncini@unipi.it

A. R. Genazzani et al. (eds.), *Menstrual Bleeding and Pain Disorders from
Adolescence to Menopause*, ISGE Series,
https://doi.org/10.1007/978-3-031-55300-4_10

histopathology (nonstructural). The classification system for fibroid location is as follows:

- Intramural myomas (FIGO type 3, 4, 5): these fibroids are located within the uterine wall, and they may be transmural and extend from the serosal to the mucosal surface.
- Submucosal myomas (FIGO type 0, 1, 2): these fibroids protrude into the uterine cavity. The extent of this protrusion is described by the FIGO/European Society of Hysteroscopy classification system [3]:

  - Type 0: completely within the endometrial cavity
  - Type 1: Extend less than 50 percent into the myometrium
  - Type 2: Extend 50 percent or more within the myometrium

- Subserosal myomas (FIGO type 6, 7): these fibroids originate from the myometrium at the serosal surface of the uterus with a broad or pedunculated base. They may be intraligamentary (i.e., extending between the folds of the broad ligament).
- Cervical myomas (FIGO type 8): these fibroids are located in the cervix.

The PALM-COEIN system adds categorization of intra-mural and subserosal myomas as well as a category that includes lesions that appear to be detached from the uterus [2]. When a myoma abuts or distorts both the endometrium and serosa, it is categorized first by the submucosal classification and then by the subserosal location, with these two numbers separated by a hyphen [4]. Considered but not yet included are the size, number, and location of the tumors longitudinally in the uterus (e.g., the fundus, lower segment, or cervix).

3   Prevalence

Uterine leiomyomas are the most common pelvic tumor in females [1, 5–7]. The actual prevalence remains unknown since studies have been conducted mainly in symptomatic patients or following surgery (i.e., hysterectomy). The incidence and prevalence of leiomyomas increase with age during the reproductive years [17]. The prevalence in postmenopausal patients is one-tenth that of premenopausal patients [8]. Moreover, while fibroids may cause heavy bleeding, bulky symptoms, or pain in the reproductive years, after menopause most fibroids will decrease in size. Leiomyomas have not been described in prepuberal girls, but they are occasionally noted in adolescents [5].

4 Pathogenesis and Risk Factors

The pathogenesis of leiomyomas is not well understood. Genetic predisposition, environmental factors, steroid hormones, and growth factors all play a role in the formation and growth of uterine fibroids. Different fibroids within the same uterus may have different etiologies and arise from different somatic mutations [9].

Two distinct components are known to contribute to leiomyoma development:

- Transformation of normal myocytes into abnormal myocytes, through somatic mutations
- Growth of abnormal myocytes into clinically apparent neoplasms

The subsequent growth of the neoplasm occurs via clonal expansion from a single cell and will likely be a better target for new therapeutic interventions [10].

5 Genetics

Uterine leiomyomas are a common phenotype with differing genotypes. There appear to be multiple different genetic pathways to phenotypic leiomyomas [11]. Most fibroids arise from somatic mutations with mediator complex subunit 12 (MED12) being by far the most common group followed by high mobility group AT-hook (HMGA1 and HMGA2) and collagen type IV, alpha-5, and alpha-6 (COL4A5 and COL4A6) [11, 12].

6 Gonadal Steroid Hormones

Gonadal steroid hormones are an important influence in leiomyoma pathogenesis. The epidemiology of leiomyomas parallels the ontogeny and life cycle changes of the reproductive hormones, estrogen and progesterone. Conventionally, estradiol has been considered the primary stimulus for fibroid growth, and studies with cell culture and animal models support this concept. However, recent findings have highlighted that progesterone appears to be the important hormone. Progesterone receptors are upregulated in leiomyomas compared with normal myometrium [13]. Although the growth of fibroids is responsive to gonadal steroids, these hormones are not necessarily responsible for the genesis of the tumors [5].

7 Parity

Parity (having one or more pregnancies extending beyond 20 weeks of gestation) decreases the chance of fibroid formation. There is also a suggestion that additional pregnancies further decrease the risk [14].

8 Early Menarche

Menarche is associated with increase of estradiol to postpubertal levels which can plausibly lead both to increased fibroid growth and early fusion of the long bone epiphyses leading to decreased height. Early menarche (<10 years old) is associated with an increased risk of developing fibroids. This may account for the early onset of disease in Black patients, in whom menarche is generally earlier than in White patients [15].

9 Obesity

BMI and weight gain exhibited a complex relation with risk uterine leiomyomata. The relationship is likely modified by other factors, such as parity, and may be more related to change in body habitus as an adult [15, 16].

10 Race/Ethnicity

The incidence rates of fibroids are typically greater in Black females than in White females. Black females compared with White females are also more likely to have clinically relevant fibroids and develop symptoms earlier [17, 18]. Differences in diet, lifestyle, psychosocial stress, perceived racism, and environmental exposures are thought to contribute to this disparity rather than race itself [19, 20].

11 Clinical Features

The majority of fibroids are asymptomatic, but many patients with myomas have significant symptoms that interfere with many aspects of their lives. These symptoms are related to the number, size, and location of the disease. Uterine leiomyomas are typically brought to medical attention due to heavy or prolonged menstrual bleeding or are found incidentally on pelvic imaging.

Symptoms are classified into three categories:

- Heavy or prolonged menstrual bleeding, the most common symptom, occurring in approximately 26–29% of all patients [5]
- Bulk-related symptoms, such as sense of abdominal fullness similar to pregnancy
- Reproductive dysfunction (i.e., infertility, miscarriage)

12 Heavy or Prolonged Menstrual Bleeding

Heavy or prolonged menstrual bleeding is the typical bleeding pattern in these women. The mechanisms of profuse menses are unclear but may include abnormalities of the uterine vasculature, impaired endometrial hemostasis, or molecular dysregulation of angiogenic factors [21]. The presence and degree of uterine bleeding are determined, in large part, by the location of the fibroid. Submucosal myomas are most frequently related to significant heavy menstrual bleeding. In addition, a study of uterine peristalsis demonstrates altered uterine contractility near submucosal fibroids; one theory is that this inhibits the usual ability of the uterus to contract during menses [22]. Intramural myomas are also commonly associated with this bleeding pattern, but subserosal fibroids are not considered a major risk for heavy menstrual bleeding [5].

13 Bulk-Related Symptoms

The myomatous uterus is enlarged and irregularly shaped causing symptoms due to pressure, such as pelvic pain or pressure (i.e., lower back pain, pelvic pain, and/or menstrual pain), urinary tract or bowel obstruction, or venous compression. Urinary symptoms including frequency, difficulty emptying the bladder, or, rarely, complete urinary obstruction may all occur in up to 60% of patients with fibroids [23]. Bladder symptoms arise when an anterior fibroid presses directly on the bladder or a posterior fibroid pushes the entire uterus forward. Likewise, fibroids that place pressure on the rectum can result in constipation.

Very large uteri may increase the thromboembolic risk due to the compression of the vena cava [24, 25]. One small study has reported thromboembolism as the presenting complaint in approximately 4% patients with an enlarged fibroid uterus [24].

14 Reproductive Dysfunction

Submucosal or intramural fibroids with an intracavitary component that distort the uterine cavity have been thought to result in difficulty conceiving a pregnancy and an increased risk of miscarriage. In addition, leiomyomas have been associated with adverse pregnancy outcomes (e.g., placental abruption, fetal growth restriction, malpresentation, and preterm labor and birth), particularly in patients with multiple fibroids, retroplacental fibroids, and size greater than 5 cm. In some patients, submucosal fibroids appear to adversely affect implantation, placentation, and ongoing pregnancy. The effects of intramural fibroids are more controversial, while fibroids that are primarily subserosal or pedunculated are unlikely to cause early pregnancy loss. The risk of pregnancy loss may be higher when there are multiple fibroids [26].

Several factors make it difficult to assess the impact of fibroids on pregnancy outcome. For example, interpretation of available evidence is limited by the heterogeneity of the study populations. Lastly, the mechanism whereby fibroids may cause adverse obstetric outcomes is not clearly understood. Most pregnant individuals with fibroids do not have any complication during pregnancy related to fibroids. When complication occurs, painful degeneration is the most common complication [27].

15 Diagnostic Evaluation

The clinical diagnosis of uterine leiomyomas is made based on a pelvic examination and pelvic ultrasound findings consistent with a uterine leiomyoma. Characteristic symptoms further support the clinical diagnosis, although many patients are asymptomatic. A definitive diagnosis by pathology evaluation is not obtained in all cases but should be pursued if there is reason to be suspicious that the uterine mass may not be a fibroid, but rather may be a uterine precancer or cancer. The differential diagnosis of uterine leiomyomas includes other conditions that cause uterine enlargement, abnormal uterine bleeding (AUB), pelvic pain, or infertility. It is important to note that leiomyomas are a common condition, and other coexisting conditions may be the etiology of the presenting symptoms.

16 History

Important information that can be elicited from the patient includes symptoms related to fibroids and their duration, severity, and impact on quality of life. Based on the bleeding pattern and risk factors, the clinician should consider the risk of endometrial hyperplasia or cancer. In addition, if there is any possibility the patient is pregnant, pregnancy testing should be performed.

Pain related to fibroids is not likely to have an acute onset, and it can also be noncyclic. In addition, pain associated with menses may also indicate other conditions, such as adenomyosis or endometriosis.

Patients should be asked about other potential pain or bulk-related symptoms, infertility, recurrent miscarriage, or obstetric complications that may be related to fibroids.

The clinician should take obstetric and gynecologic history including prior history of uterine fibroids, history of pelvic pain, and relevant medical and surgical history, including those that are part of the differential diagnosis or may exacerbate the symptoms of a pelvic mass, pelvic pain, or abnormal uterine bleeding. It should include also risk factors for uterine malignancies other than endometrial carcinoma (sarcoma, carcinosarcoma).

17 Physical Examination

The physical examination includes an abdominal and pelvic examination. The abdominal examination should include palpation for a pelvic-abdominal mass. Large fibroid uteri can be palpated abdominally. The level of the uterine fundus should be noted. The size is described in terms of the fundal height in the superior-inferior axis in comparison to a gravid uterus.

A thorough pelvic examination is performed. On bimanual pelvic examination, the size, contour, and mobility should be noted. An enlarged, mobile uterus with an irregular contour is consistent with a leiomyomatous uterus. An enlarged uterus that is fixed raises suspicion of an inflammatory process or malignancy.

18 Laboratory Testing

Laboratory testing does not have a role in the diagnosis but is important in evaluating for other associated conditions, including pregnancy, anemia, endometrial hyperplasia, or carcinoma (i.e., endometrial biopsy).

19 Imaging and Endoscopy

Pelvic ultrasound is the first-line study used to evaluate uterine fibroids, based on the ability to visualize genital tract structures and cost-effectiveness. Fibroids are seen on pelvic ultrasound as well-circumscribed round masses, hypoechoic, frequently with shadowing. Precise localization of fibroids is limited in larger uteri or when there are many tumors [5].

Diagnostic hysteroscopy is useful for visualizing endometrial cavity. This technique allows evaluation for submucosal or protruding myometrial fibroids and can characterize the extent of protrusion. However, when the fibroid abuts the endometrium or protrudes into the myometrium, the depth of penetration cannot be ascertained hysteroscopically.

Hysterosalpingograms can also sometimes show the distortion of the endometrial cavity in those patients needing assessment of fallopian tube patency for fertility.

Additional imaging can be necessary when complex intervention is planned or malignant disease is suspected (i.e., magnetic resonance imaging, contrast-enhanced ultrasound).

20 Treatment Overview

Uterine fibroids can be entirely asymptomatic. However, many patients will present with symptoms including abnormal uterine bleeding, pressure or bulk symptoms, fertility issues, and/or pain that warrants treatment. The patient's desire for immediate or future pregnancy has to be assessed prior to choosing any treatment as the therapies have differing impacts on fertility.

20.1 Patient Not Desiring Fertility

For patients who do not desire fertility, treatment is aimed at symptom reduction.

When there is an underlying condition, its treatment can correct the AUB or make further treatment more effective.

First-tier treatment of heavy menstrual bleeding, which is a common presenting symptom in patients with fibroids, includes hysteroscopic fibroid resection, if the fibroids are in an appropriate anatomic location, or medical treatment for those with fibroids in locations not amenable to hysteroscopic resection.

Hysteroscopic myomectomy is on outpatient procedure with rapid recovery, a low risk of complications compared with abdominal procedures, rapid improvement in quality of life, and low risk for uterine rupture in subsequent pregnancy [28].

Combined estrogen-progestin contraceptives (oral contraceptive pills, vaginal ring, or transdermal patch) are the most common medical therapy utilized in patients with all other types of fibroids who do not desire pregnancy [29]. For patients who cannot use or do not want estrogen-containing contraceptives, progestin-releasing intrauterine devices (IUDs) are the main progestin-only contraceptive for fibroid-related heavy menstrual bleeding, although supporting data are mainly observational [30].

Effective second-tier medical treatments for fibroid-associated HMB are gonadotropin-releasing hormone (GnRH) agonist and antagonists [31]. Uterine artery embolization is a minimally invasive treatment option that treats bot bleeding and bulk symptoms [32].

For patients who do not desire future fertility and have persistent fibroid-related symptoms or who desire surgical treatment, main options include hysterectomy and myomectomy. Hysterectomy involves removal of the uterine corpus, including the fibroids, while myomectomy removes only the fibroids and leaves the uterus in situ.

Hysterectomy eliminates both the risk of new fibroids forming and all types of abnormal uterine bleeding, and it improves quality of life [33]. However, hysterectomy has also been associated with long-term morbidity with and without bilateral oophorectomy.

20.2 Patients Desiring Fertility

Most medical therapies for uterine fibroids preclude conception, cause adverse effects when employed long-term, and result in rapid symptom rebound when discontinued. For patients with heavy menstrual bleeding and a submucosal fibroid or fibroids (FIGO type 0, 1 or some type 2), hysteroscopic myomectomy is appropriate. For patients who desire pregnancy and present with bulk symptoms, treatment can be represented by myomectomy via either laparoscopy (with or without robotic assistance) or an open abdominal incision. Laparoscopic myomectomy compared with open abdominal myomectomy presents decreased morbidity and a shorter recovery. However, laparoscopic technique may be limited by characteristics of myomas and surgical expertise [34].

References

1. Baird DD, Dunson DB, Hill MC, Cousins D, Schectman JM. High cumulative incidence of uterine leiomyoma in black and white women: ultrasound evidence. Am J Obstet Gynecol. 2003;188(1):100–7. https://doi.org/10.1067/mob.2003.99.
2. Munro MG, Critchley HOD, Fraser IS. The FIGO classification of causes of abnormal uterine bleeding in the reproductive years. Fertil Steril. 2011;95(7):2204. https://doi.org/10.1016/j.fertnstert.2011.03.079.
3. Wamsteker K, Emanuel MH, de Kruif JH. Transcervical hysteroscopic resection of submucous fibroids for abnormal uterine bleeding: results regarding the degree of intramural extension. Obstet Gynecol. 1993;82(5):736–40.
4. Munro MG, Critchley HOD, Broder MS, Fraser IS. FIGO classification system (PALM-COEIN) for causes of abnormal uterine bleeding in nongravid women of reproductive age. Int J Gynecol Obstet. 2011;113(1):3–13. https://doi.org/10.1016/j.ijgo.2010.11.011.
5. Stewart E. Uterine fibroids (leiomyomas): epidemiology, clinical features, diagnosis, and natural history. UpToDate®; 2021. p. 1–51. https://www-uptodate-com.ezaccess.library.uitm.edu.my/contents/uterine-fibroids-leiomyomas-epidemiology-clinical-features-diagnosis-and-natural-history?search=leiomyoma&source=search_result&selectedTitle=1~150&usage_type=default&display_rank=1
6. Buttram VC, Reiter RC. Uterine leiomyomata: etiology, symptomatology, and management. Fertil Steril. 1981;36(4):433–45.
7. Marshall LM, Spiegelman D, Barbieri RL, et al. Variation in the incidence of uterine leiomyoma among premenopausal women by age and race. Obstet Gynecol. 1997;90(6):967–73. https://doi.org/10.1016/S0029-7844(97)00534-6.

8. Paramsothy P, Harlow SD, Greendale GA, et al. Bleeding patterns during the menopausal transition in the multi-ethnic Study of Women's Health Across the Nation (SWAN): a prospective cohort study. BJOG An Int J Obstet Gynaecol. 2014;121(12):1564–73. https://doi.org/10.1111/1471-0528.12768.

9. Peddada SD, Laughlin SK, Miner K, et al. Growth of uterine leiomyomata among premenopausal black and white women. Proc Natl Acad Sci USA. 2008;105(50):19887–92. https://doi.org/10.1073/pnas.0808188105.

10. Hashimoto K, Azuma C, Kamiura S, Kimura T, Nobunaga T, Kanai T, Sawada M, Noguchi SSF. Clonal determination of uterine leiomyomas by analyzing differential inactivation of the X-chromosome-linked phosphoglycerokinase gene. Gynecol Obs Invest. 1995;40(3):204.

11. Mehine M, Kaasinen E, Mäkinen N, et al. Characterization of uterine leiomyomas by whole-genome sequencing. N Engl J Med. 2013;369(1):43–53. https://doi.org/10.1056/nejmoa1302736.

12. Mehine M, Mäkinen N, Heinonen HR, Aaltonen LA, Vahteristo P. Genomics of uterine leiomyomas: insights from high-throughput sequencing. Fertil Steril. 2014;102(3):621–9. https://doi.org/10.1016/j.fertnstert.2014.06.050.

13. Ishikawa H, Ishi K, Ann Serna V, Kakazu R, Bulun SE, Kurita T. Progesterone is essential for maintenance and growth of uterine leiomyoma. Endocrinology. 2010;151(6):2433–42. https://doi.org/10.1210/en.2009-1225.

14. Marshall LM, Spiegelman D, Goldman MB, et al. A prospective study of reproductive factors and oral contraceptive use in relation to the risk of uterine leiomyomata. Fertil Steril. 1998;70(3):432–9. https://doi.org/10.1016/S0015-0282(98)00208-8.

15. Wise LA, Palmer JR, Harlow BL, et al. Reproductive factors, hormonal contraception, and risk of uterine leiomyomata in African–American women: a prospective study. Am J Epidemiol. 2004;159(2):113–23. https://doi.org/10.1093/aje/kwh016.

16. Wise LA, Palmer JR, Spiegelman D, et al. Influence of body size and body fat distribution on risk of uterine leiomyomata in U.S. black women. Epidemiology. 2005;16(3):346–54. https://doi.org/10.1097/01.ede.0000158742.11877.99.

17. Harmon QE, Actkins KV, Baird DD. Fibroid prevalence-still so much to learn. JAMA Netw Open. 2023;6(5):E2312682. https://doi.org/10.1001/jamanetworkopen.2023.12682.

18. Madrigano J. 基因的改变 NIH Public Access. Occup Env Med. 2008;23(1):1–7.

19. Vines AI, Ta M, Esserman DA. The association between self-reported major life events and the presence of uterine fibroids. Womens Health Issues. 2010;20(4):294–8.

20. Boynton-Jarrett R, Rich-Edwards JW, Jun HJ, Hibert ENWR. Abuse in childhood and risk of uterine leiomyoma: the role of emotional support in biologic resilience. Epidemiology. 2011;22(1):6–14.

21. Puri K, Famuyide AO, Erwin PJ, Stewart EAL-TS. Submucosal fibroids and the relation to heavy menstrual bleeding and anemia. Am J Obs Gynecol. 2014;210(1):38.e1–7. Epub 2013 Sep 28

22. Deligdish LLM. Endometrial changes associated with myomata of the uterus. J Clin Pathol. 1970;23(8):676–80.

23. Lee DW, Gibson TB, Carls GS, Ozminkowski RJ, Wang SSE. Uterine fibroid treatment patterns in a population of insured women. Fertil Steril. 2009;91(2):566–74. Epub 2008 Mar 4

24. Fletcher HM, Wharfe G, Williams NP, Gordon-Strachan GJP. Renal impairment as a complication of uterine fibroids: a retrospective hospital-based study. J Obs Gynaecol. 2013;33(4):394–8.

25. Shiota M, Kotani Y, Umemoto M, Tobiume T, Tsuritani M, Shimaoka MHH. Deep-vein thrombosis is associated with large uterine fibroids. Tohoku J Exp Med. 2011;224(2):87.

26. Benson CB, Chow JS, Chang-Lee W, Hill JA 3rd, Doubilet PM. Outcome of pregnancies in women with uterine leiomyomas identified by sonography in the first trimester. J Clin Ultrasound. 2001;29(5):261.

27. Segars JH, Parrott EC, Nagel JD, Guo XC, Gao X, Birnbaum LS, Pinn VWDD. Proceedings from the Third National Institutes of Health International Congress on Advances in Uterine Leiomyoma Research: comprehensive review, conference summary and future recommendations. Hum Reprod Update. 2014;20(3):309–33. Epub 2014 Jan 8
28. Marret H, Fritel X, Ouldamer L, Bendifallah S, Brun JL, De Jesus I, Derrien J, Giraudet G, Kahn V, Koskas M, Legendre G, Lucot JP, Niro J, Panel P, Pelage JP, Fernandez HC, CNGOF French College of Gynecology and Obstetrics. Therapeutic management of uterine fibroid tumors: updated French guidelines. Eur J Obs Gynecol Reprod Biol. 2012;165(2):156–64. Epub 2012 Aug 29
29. Yao Z, Shen X, Capodanno I, et al. Validation of rat endometriosis model by using raloxifene as a positive control for the evaluation of novel SERM compounds. J Investig Surg. 2005;18(4):177–83. https://doi.org/10.1080/08941930591004412.
30. Sangkomkamhang US, Lumbiganon P. Progestogens or progestogen-releasing intrauterine systems for uterine fibroids (other than preoperative medical therapy). Cochrane Database Syst Rev. 2020;11:CD008994. Epub 2020 Nov 23
31. Lethaby A, Puscasiu LVB. Preoperative medical therapy before surgery for uterine fibroids. Cochrane Database Syst Rev. 2017;11:CD000547. Epub 2017 Nov 15
32. Yoon JK, Han K, Kim MD, Kim GM, Kwon JH, Won JYLD. Five-year clinical outcomes of uterine artery embolization for symptomatic leiomyomas: an analysis of risk factors for reintervention. Eur J Radiol. 2018. Epub 2018 Oct 28;109:83.
33. Kuppermann M, Learman LA, Schembri M, Gregorich SE, Jackson RA, Jacoby A, Lewis JWA. Contributions of hysterectomy and uterus-preserving surgery to health-related quality of life. Obstet Gynecol. 2013;122(1):15.
34. Parker WHRI. Patient selection for laparoscopic myomectomy. J Am Assoc Gynecol Laparosc. 1994;2(1):23.

Endometrial Malignancy and Hyperplasia as Causes of Abnormal Uterine Bleeding

Catrambone Ilaria, Andrea Giannini, and Tommaso Simoncini

1 Introduction

Abnormal uterine bleeding (AUB) is a common disorder defined as heavy uterine bleeding or intermenstrual uterine bleeding in the reproductive years [1] or any kind of uterine bleeding in the postmenopause. Abnormal uterine bleeding is usually associated with a benign condition but can be a major symptom of endometrial hyperplasia or endometrial carcinoma [2]. For this reason, all possible causes of uterine bleeding in women of childbearing age and women after menopause should be investigated.

Abnormal uterine bleeding can depend on various causes, and there are various risk factors, which mostly depend on the woman's age. In the reproductive years, abnormal uterine bleeding may result from pregnancy, miscarriage, ectopic pregnancy, hormonal disorders, cervical or endometrial polyps, and, more rarely, endometrial hyperplasia or even carcinoma [3]. In contrast, in the postmenopausal age, the most common cause of abnormal uterine bleeding is the thinning of the tissues that line the uterus or vagina, followed by uterine polyps. Less common but more critical causes for women's health are endometrial hyperplasia, with or without atypia, and endometrial cancer.

C. Ilaria · A. Giannini (✉) · T. Simoncini
Department of Clinical and Experimental Medicine, Division of Obstetrics and Gynecology, University of Pisa, Pisa, Italy
e-mail: andrea.giannini@unipi.it; tommso.simoncini@unipi.it

A. R. Genazzani et al. (eds.), *Menstrual Bleeding and Pain Disorders from Adolescence to Menopause*, ISGE Series,
https://doi.org/10.1007/978-3-031-55300-4_11

2   FIGO Classification System

FIGO (International Federation of Gynecology and Obstetrics) has developed two AUB classification systems to standardize definitions, nomenclature, and underlying categories of etiology [4, 5]:

- System 1, which is based on a standardized definition of abnormal uterine bleeding in childbearing years
- System 2 (the PALM-COEIN system), which contains the most common causes of abnormal uterine bleeding

System 1 is based on the main characteristics of menstrual cycles, such as duration, frequency, and quantity; in fact, it divides abnormal uterine bleeding into heavy menstrual bleeding (HMB, i.e., excessive menstrual bleeding affecting the quality of life of women); bleeding between periods; and breakthrough bleeding (BTB, which can occur with hormonal drugs such as birth control pills).

System 2 summarizes the most common causes of abnormal uterine bleeding under the acronym PALM-COEIN and divides them into structural causes (PALM) and non-structural causes (COEIN), which will be described in detail below. PALM: polyps, adenomyosis, leiomyoma, malignancy, hyperplasia. COEIN: coagulopathy, hormonal dysfunction, iatrogenic cause, not yet classified.

2.1   *Polyps (AUB—P)*

Endometrial polyps can be single or multiple lesions, a few millimeters or several centimeters long, and their morphology can be sessile or pedunculated. The main risk factors for the development of endometrial polyps are older age, hypertension, obesity, treatment with tamoxifen, and any conditions that promote hypoestrogenism (e.g., polycystic ovary syndrome, obesity, late menopause, early menarche) [6]. Polyps can be asymptomatic, but when they do produce symptoms, the most common is abnormal uterine bleeding, and in some cases, they can be associated with infertility. Additionally, although rare, polyps can be associated with malignant lesions, with an estimated prevalence of 3.4% to 4.9% in postmenopausal age and 1.1% before menopause. The main risk factors for transformation into malignant lesions are advanced age, the presence of abnormal uterine bleeding, and obesity. Diagnosis of endometrial polyps is mainly based on pelvic ultrasound, which identifies the polyp and describes its characteristics (size, whether it is sessile or pedunculated, etc.). After identification and description of the polyp by ultrasound, it may be necessary to resort to hysteroscopy, which makes it possible to carry out a targeted biopsy, to make a histological diagnosis excluding malignant lesions. The therapeutic management of endometrial polyps essentially depends on the woman's age and its clinical manifestations. Indeed, if the woman is of reproductive years and the polyp is asymptomatic, it is possible to allow watchful waiting with frequent observation. Instead, in postmenopausal women with endometrial polyps causing AUB, it is necessary to intervene with hysteroscopically guided polypectomy, through which it is possible to remove the lesion and make a histological diagnosis.

2.2   Adenomyosis (AUB—A)

Adenomyosis is a benign disorder in which endometrial glands and stroma exist in the myometrium. It is usually associated with increasing age and may coexist with uterine fibroids. In addition, adenomyosis can be focal or widespread and may be more difficult to diagnose when co-existing with fibroids [5].

2.3   Malignancy (AUB—M)

This group includes endometrial hyperplasia with or without atypia and endometrial cancer, which will be described in detail below.

2.4   Coagulopathy (AUB—C)

Coagulopathy occurs in 13% of women with AUB. Most of these women have von Willebrand's disease. Until now, anticoagulants and antiplatelet drugs were considered part of "AUB-C" [5].

2.5   Ovulatory (AUB—O)

Anovulatory cycles, along with changes in menstrual frequency, may contribute to AUB through the unopposed effects of estrogen on the endometrium. This is observed at the extremes of reproductive age. However, with endocrinopathy, the hypothalamus-pituitary-ovary axis can also be affected. The latter includes factors such as obesity, anorexia, weight loss, mental stress, and intense exercise, as well as polycystic ovary syndrome (PCOS), hyperprolactinemia, and hypothyroidism. Concomitant ovulatory dysfunction in women with uterine fibroids may exacerbate the menstrual loss [5].

2.6 Endometrial (AUB—E)

AUB occurring in association with a structurally normal uterus with regular menstrual cycles without signs of coagulopathy may have an underlying endometrial cause. Endometrial function related to menstruation and its disorders has not yet been fully studied and remains an active area of scientific research. AUB—E can occur in many women with AUB, but the lack of specific tests or clinically available biomarkers means that a true test for the condition is not yet available. Diagnosis, therefore, depends on careful history taking and the exclusion of other participants [5].

2.7 Iatrogenic (AUB—I)

Iatrogenic causes of AUB include exogenous therapies that can cause unscheduled endometrial bleeding. It is usually associated with interventions that affect ovarian steroid secretion, such as continuous estrogen or progesterone therapy (systemic or intrauterine routes) or gonadotropin-releasing hormone (GnRH) agonists and aromatase inhibitors. Selective estrogen receptor modulators (SERMs) and, rarely, selective progesterone receptor modulators (SPRMs) can cause AUB by acting directly on the endometrium [5].

2.8 Not Otherwise Classified (AUB-N)

Inevitably, there are rare or ill-defined pathologies that do not fit easily into the previously described categories. Examples include arteriovenous malformations, endometrial pseudoaneurysms, myometrial enlargement, and chronic endometritis [5].

3 Endometrial Hyperplasia With or Without Atypia

Endometrial hyperplasia represents an abnormal proliferation of endometrial glands leading to an increased gland-to-stroma ratio relative to endometrium from the proliferative phase of the cycle. Proliferating glands in endometrial hyperplasia may vary greatly in size and shape, and cytologic atypia may be present [7, 8]. There are two types of endometrial hyperplasia: hyperplasia without atypia and hyperplasia with atypia (atypical hyperplasia or endometrial intraepithelial neoplasia, EIN). The clinical significance of a diagnosis of endometrial hyperplasia correlates with the risk of long-term progression to endometrial cancer; indeed, atypical endometrial hyperplasia is thought to be a precursor to endometrioid endometrial carcinoma, as both share a similar profile of genetic alterations and monoclonal growth. Up to 60% of patients with endometrial hyperplasia with atypia have already developed or will develop invasive endometrial cancer, whereas hyperplasia without atypia rarely progresses to endometrial cancer (1–3%). In some cases, endometrial hyperplasia with atypia is a marker of concurrent cancer (i.e., the simultaneous presence of endometrial hyperplasia with atypia and endometrial carcinoma) [7]. For these reasons, endometrial tissue sampling should be performed in all women suspected of having endometrial hyperplasia [9].

The main symptom of endometrial hyperplasia is abnormal uterine bleeding [8], and the main factor stimulating the development of hyperplasia is excess estrogen. In fact, the main risk factor is anovulation (e.g., a common risk factor of hyperplasia with atypia in reproductive age is polycystic ovary syndrome and postmenopausal obesity). When treating a patient with endometrial hyperplasia, it is first necessary to determine the risk of progression to endometrial cancer and whether there is concurrent cancer [10]. The risk of progression to endometrial cancer varies depending on whether it is hyperplasia without atypia (in this case the risk of progression is 4.6% in 20 years) or hyperplasia with atypia or intraepithelial neoplasia (in this case the risk of progression is 28%) [11]. In terms of concurrent carcinoma, the literature describes a prevalence between 17% and 52%. In the case of endometrial hyperplasia without atypia, the first-line therapy is a medical approach, which can be based on estrogen-progestogen or progestogen-only drugs, oral or vaginal. A minimum treatment duration of 6 months is generally required to induce regression of endometrial hyperplasia without atypia. Follow-up is based on endometrial sampling taken every 3–6 months to ensure that no disease progression occurs during treatment. Patients who do not respond after 12 months of treatment will rarely experience a response thereafter, and a change in treatment modality should be considered. Surgical treatment should be reserved for patients who do not wish to preserve their fertility and who have progressed to atypical hyperplasia or carcinoma during follow-up. However, the surgical approach for endometrial hyperplasia without atypia should be total hysterectomy with salpingectomy, with or without bilateral oophorectomy [9].

In the case of endometrial hyperplasia with atypia, the first-line therapy is hysterectomy with adnexectomy or salpingectomy, and a minimally invasive approach is preferred [9]. A particular case is represented by a woman with endometrial hyperplasia in reproductive years who wants to preserve her fertility: in this case, it is possible to carry out hormone therapy based on progestins (oral or local), aromatase inhibitors, or gonadotropin-releasing hormone agonists [9] and careful follow-up [7]. The follow-up should be done every 3 months until at least two negative specimens are obtained. Patients who develop cancer progression during follow-up, whose hyperplasia does not resolve after 12 months of medical treatment, or who relapse after discontinuation of progestogen therapy, or who continue to experience abnormal uterine bleeding despite treatment, or who refuse endometrial monitoring or medical treatment, should undergo definitive surgical treatment [9].

4 Endometrial Cancer

Endometrial cancer is the sixth most common cancer in women, and in most cases, its main or only symptom is abnormal uterine bleeding [12]. Usually AUB occurs at a relatively early stage of the disease, and it can be considered a good trigger for evaluation of the endometrial cavity [13].

There are two types of endometrial carcinoma, type I and type II, which differ from an epidemiological, histopathological, prognostic, and therapeutic point of view. Type I endometrioid carcinoma is estrogen-dependent, is more common, and generally has a lower recurrence rate and a more favorable prognosis (with an 85% overall 5-year survival rate) because it is usually confined to the uterus at the time of diagnosis and is usually low-grade (FIGO grade 1 or 2) cancer. EIN is considered a precursor to type I cancer, which is more common in younger, obese women. Type II non-endometrioid carcinoma is not estrogen-dependent and is considered high grade by definition, and it generally has a poorer prognosis (with an overall 5-year survival rate of 55%) and a higher recurrence rate [14]. This group includes clear cell carcinoma and serous carcinoma [12], but mixed cell, undifferentiated, neuroendocrine, and carcinosarcomas also belong to this group. The main risk factors for the development of endometrial cancer are obesity, tamoxifen therapy, and chronic exposure to hypoestrogenism, both endogenous (early menarche, late menopause, chronic anovulation, nulliparity, infertility) and exogenous (like hormone replacement therapy); and there may also be a genetic predisposition (Lynch syndrome or Cowden syndrome). The most common symptom is abnormal uterine bleeding, but, especially in the more advanced stages of the disease, women may also have abdominal pain, vaginal discharge, abdominal distension, changes in bowel or bladder function, and dyspnea because of pleural effusion [14]. FIGO staging of endometrial cancer is the most commonly used and recognizes four tumor stages, based on myometrial infiltration and the local and distant extent of the disease (Table 1). To stage the disease, a gynecological examination and transvaginal ultrasound are required to assess tumor volume, myometrial infiltration, cervical involvement, and the presence of ovarian disease [12]. The diagnosis is confirmed by a biopsy performed by hysteroscopy or dilation and curettage. Diagnostic methods such as magnetic resonance (MR) or computed tomography (CT) can also be used to exclude metastases [14].

Table 1 In the case of early-stage disease (FIGO stage I), the first-line treatment is surgical access (by laparotomy, laparoscopy, or robotic) with total hysterectomy, bilateral adnexectomy, and with or without lymphadenectomy [12]. Regarding the role of lymphadenectomy, it is important during surgery to assess pelvic lymph nodes and remove enlarged lymph nodes to exclude metastases, even for women in whom uterine confinement is suspected, as this may determine the need for adjuvant treatment with radiotherapy and/or chemotherapy and provide important prognostic information. In young women who wish to preserve their fertility, it is possible to carry out a conservative approach based on progestogen treatment, provided that certain characteristics are present, i.e., that the tumor has an endometrioid histotype,

Table 1 FIGO classification system 2009 [12]

Stage I	Tumor confined to the body of the uterus
IA	No infiltration or infiltration of <½ myometrium
IB	Infiltration >½ myometrium
Stage II	Tumor extended to the cervical stroma but not outside the uterus
Stage III	Local or regional extension
IIIA	Extension to the uterine serosa or ovaries
III B	Extension to the vagina or parameters
III C	Extension to pelvic or lumbo-aortic lymph nodes
IIIC1	Pelvic lymph nodes positive
III C2	Lumbo-aortic lymph nodes positive, regardless of the pelvic ones
Stage IV	Extension to the bladder or intestinal mucosa or distant metastases
IVA	Extension to the bladder or intestinal mucosa
IVB	Distant metastases

that it is well differentiated, and that invasion of the myometrium is minimal or absent. This type of pharmacological treatment is temporary and aimed only at achieving pregnancy and must be discontinued as the disease progresses. In stage II, the first-line treatment is surgery, but a radical hysterectomy is necessary. On the contrary, in the more advanced stages (stage III and IV FIGO), the surgical approach only has a palliative role, and chemotherapy is the first-line treatment [12]. In patients in whom surgery is not possible (e.g., patients with unresectable disease or with significant medical comorbidities), radiotherapy and/or chemotherapy is the preferred treatment. Risk stratification should be done to decide what kind of follow-up care should be done or if the patient needs adjuvant therapy. Low-risk endometrial cancer includes women with grade 1 or 2 endometrioid histology limited to the endometrium (FIGO stage IA). In this case, there is a small risk of recurrence, so adjuvant therapy is not recommended. Intermediate-risk endometrial cancer is defined as cancer confined to the uterus but invading the myometrium (FIGO stage IA or IB) or cancer with cervical stromal invasion (FIGO stage II). This intermediate-risk group can be further divided into high and low intermediate-risk groups based on age and some pathologic factors (such as the presence of deep myometrial invasion or the presence of invasion of the lymph vascular space). For low intermediate-risk endometrial cancer, observation only is recommended, and radiation therapy should be considered in high intermediate-risk disease as it may reduce the risk of local recurrence [14].

5 Diagnosis and Management of Abnormal Uterine Bleeding

If a woman comes to clinic with abnormal uterine bleeding, first of all, a complete medical history should be collected to rule out pregnancy, the use of medications (e.g., oral contraceptives), and IUDs. A medical history can also help you understand how long the uterine bleeding has lasted, how it relates to weight gain or loss, gender, drug use, and the presence of other symptoms. The second step is a gynecological examination with speculum examination if possible. A complete gynecologic examination is helpful to rule out nongynecological causes of bleeding (e.g., clotting disorders) and nonuterine causes of bleeding (including evaluation of the vulva, vagina, and cervix). The third step is based on laboratory tests and imaging. Laboratory tests include pregnancy tests, hormone levels, liver and thyroid function tests, and coagulation tests. Transvaginal pelvic ultrasound is the main method for diagnosing uterine pathologies such as endometrial polyps, endometrial hypertrophy, adnexal masses, and polycystic ovarian syndrome [2]. If the ultrasound diagnosis is inconclusive, MRI or CT can be used. In most cases of women with AUB, to complete the diagnosis, it is also necessary to resort to invasive tests, such as endometrial sampling and hysteroscopy. Endometrial cancer is often diagnosed with endometrial sampling by hysteroscopy or with in-office endometrial biopsy, curettage, or targeted endometrial biopsy [15].

6 Endometrial Sampling

In the UK, NICE recommended endometrial sampling for women over 45 years of age with persistent breakthrough bleeding or treatment failure. The RCOG guidelines published in 2008 emphasized this, except for lowering the sampling age to 40 years in the setting of treatment failure.

Because of the significant increase in endometrial cancer, endometrial sampling was recommended in women over 40 years of age with HMB who had risk factors for malignant transformation, such as obesity and PCOS. In 2012, the American College of Obstetricians and Gynecologists (ACOG), in their Practice Bulletin, acknowledged "the primary role of endometrial sampling in patients with AUB is to determine if carcinoma or pre-malignant lesions are present." Furthermore, the Bulletin states that endometrial biopsy has "high overall accuracy in diagnosing endometrial cancer when an adequate specimen is obtained and when the endometrial process is global" (>50% of the uterine cavity surface). Therefore, these tests are now considered an endpoint when they show carcinoma or atypical complex hyperplasia The most accurate method of obtaining histological specimens is not yet known, for many years dilation and curettage (D&C) was the method of choice, but all or part of the focal lesion may remain in the uterine cavity after D&C in women with focal lesions in growth. Alternatively, hysteroscopy offers the advantage of distinguishing between normal and abnormal endometrium due to direct visualization of the uterine cavity and targeted biopsies [16].

7   Role of Hysteroscopy

Hysteroscopy is a procedure to examine the inside of the uterus. This is done by passing transcervically a thin telescope-like device called a hysteroscope, which is fitted with a small camera. This procedure is performed without general or regional anesthesia. Vaginoscopy is the recommended technique, and a miniature hystero-scope (3.5 mm or smaller) should be used [17]. Hysteroscopy remains the gold standard for the detection of uterine bleeding and is particularly useful clinically in patients with focal lesions and/or recurrent menopausal bleeding. Office hysteros-copy has been useful in the preoperative setting to inform malignant risk and to predict cervical metastases of endometrial adenocarcinoma. Advantages of hyster-oscopy include direct visualization of the endometrial cavity and hysteroscopy-guided biopsy. The procedural risks of this method are minimal and include cervical injury, bleeding, and fluid overload due to intraperitoneal absorption of the expand-ing medium. Hysteroscopy with or without biopsy would be appropriate in women with any postmenopausal bleeding when the endometrial thickness is >4 mm. An incidental finding of a thicker endometrium need not warrant investigation although on a case by case basis, if deemed high risk (marked obesity, history of PCOS, unopposed estrogen, etc.), then evaluation may be appropriate.

8   Hysteroscopy Can Also Have a Surgical Role, in Fact, It Can Remove Endometrial Lesions

When performing a hysteroscopy, it is important to choose the most appropriate form of distention media according to the purpose of the hysteroscopy [18]: if a diagnostic hysteroscopy is performed, a simple saline solution can be used, which is very cheap and allows a clear view, while if it is necessary to perform an operative hysteroscopy, it is necessary to use electronic fluid management systems that allow the dilatation of the uterine cavity and the control of the intrauterine pressure. However, biopsies can be performed using the classic punch biopsy technique, which allows the removal of small tissue fragments and does not allow targeted biopsy of the lesion. Alternatively, the biopsy can be performed with scissors or a bipolar electrode, particularly effective in cases of atrophic endometrium where punch biopsy is more difficult. In a study performing blind endometrial sampling in 65 patients with known carcinoma before their hysterectomy, results assessed that 11/65 cancers were missed with a sensitivity of only 83%. Causes of a low sample include cervical stenosis, uterine prolapse, focal endometrial pathology (e.g., uter-ine polyps and submucosal fibroids), and endometrial atrophy. If a histological diagnosis of the sample is inadequate, gynecologists are sometimes unsure whether to proceed with further invasive studies for fear that cancer will disappear. The hysteroscopy-guided biopsy is a more sensitive, specific, and precise technique that reduces the number of ultrasounds and follow-up visits. According to NICE guidelines [17] office, hysteroscopy is recommended instead of pelvic ultrasonography for investigation of suspicion of submucosal fibroids, polyps, or endometrial pathology. It is an efficient and safe technique with a low risk of complications, pain, and anxiety for most people [19].

References

1. Davidson BR. Abnormal uterine bleeding during the reproductive years. J Midwifery Womens Health. 2012;57(3):248–54.
2. Clarke MA. Risk assessment of endometrial cancer and endometrial intraepithelial neoplasia in women with abnormal bleeding and implications for clinical management algorithms. Am J Obstet Gynecol. 2020;223(4):549.
3. Kaunitz AM. Abnormal uterine bleeding in reproductive-age women. JAMA. 2019;321(21):2126–7.
4. Munro MG. Figo-sistema di classificazione (palm-coein) delle cause di sanguinamento uterino anomalo in donne non gravide e in età riproduttiva. Giornale italiano di ostetricia e ginecologia. 2011;33(5):289–303.
5. Whitaker L, Critchley HO. Abnormal uterine bleeding. Best Pract Res Clin Obstet Gynaecol. 2016;34:54–65.
6. Vitale SG. Endometrial polyps. An evidence-based diagnosis and management guide. Eur J Obstet Gynecol Reprod Biol. 2021;260:70–7.
7. Armstrong AJ. Diagnosis and management of endometrial hyperplasia. J Minim Invasive Gynecol. 2012;19(5):562–71.
8. Sanderson PA. New concepts for an old problem: the diagnosis of endometrial hyperplasia. Hum Reprod Update. 2017;23(2):232–54.
9. Auclair M-HE. Guideline no. 390-classification and management of endometrial hyperplasia. J Obstet Gynaecol Canada. 2019;41(12):1789–800.
10. Giede KC. Significance of concurrent endometrial cancer in women with a preoperative diagnosis of atypical endometrial hyperplasia. J Obstet Gynaecol Canada. 2008;30(10):896–901.
11. Trimble CL. Concurrent endometrial carcinoma in women with a biopsy diagnosis of atypical endometrial hyperplasia: a Gynecologic Oncology Group Study. Cancer. 2006;106(4):812–9.
12. Linee guida aiom. Neoplasie dell'utero: endometrio e cervice.
13. Kimura TE. Abnormal uterine bleeding and prognosis of endometrial cancer. Int J Gynecol Obstet. 2004;85(2):145–50.
14. Passarello K, Kurian S, Villanueva V. Endometrial cancer: an overview of pathophysiology, management, and care. Semin Oncol Nurs. 2019;35:157–65.
15. Larish AE. Impact of hysteroscopy on course of disease in high-risk endometrial carcinoma. Int J Gynecol Cancer. 2020;30(10):1513.
16. Bourdel NE. Sampling in atypical endometrial hyperplasia: which method results in the lowest underestimation of endometrial cancer? A systematic review and meta-analysis. J Minim Invasive Gynecol. 2016;23(5):692–701.
17. Heavy menstrual bleeding. S.l.:NICE.
18. Haimovich S, Tanvir T. A mini-review of office hysteroscopic techniques for endometrial tissue sampling in postmenopausal bleeding. J Midlife Health. 2021;12(1):21.
19. Best practice in outpatient hysteroscopy. Guideline, rcog/bsge joint. 2011.

Unique Issues in Oncological Patients: From Amenorrhea to Fertility Preservation

Marta Caretto, Martina Benvenuti, and Tommaso Simoncini

1 Introduction

Cancer is an important cause of morbidity and mortality worldwide, with 18.1 million new cases and 9.6 million cancer deaths worldwide in 2018 [1]. Breast cancer is the most common female cancer worldwide, followed by colorectal cancer in high-income countries and cervical cancer in low- and middle-income countries.

Worldwide, there were about 2.1 million newly diagnosed female breast cancer cases in 2018, accounting for almost one in four cancer cases among women. Approximately 20% of new breast cancer diagnoses occur in women under age 45, with almost all requiring chemotherapy and adjuvant endocrine therapy. With earlier detection and improved treatments, particularly in high-income countries, women are living longer after a cancer diagnosis [2].

At the time of diagnosis, a significant proportion of young women experience unique treatment and survivorship issues centering on treatment-related amenorrhea, including fertility preservation and management of ovarian function as endocrine therapy. Considering the rising trend in delaying childbearing and the higher number of patients who have not completed their family planning at the time of diagnosis, the demand for fertility preservation and information about the feasibility and safety of pregnancy following treatment completion is expected to increase [3].

One of the main issues that influence patients' quality of life after adjuvant chemotherapy is the risk for infertility [4]. Chemotherapy-induced amenorrhea (CIA) is a well-known toxicity after chemotherapy in young cancer patients that has traditionally referred as a marker of infertility. The majority of young cancer patients

M. Caretto (✉) · M. Benvenuti · T. Simoncini
Department of Clinical and Experimental Medicine, Division of Obstetrics and Gynecology, University of Pisa, Pisa, Italy
e-mail: tommaso.simoncini@unipi.it

A. R. Genazzani et al. (eds.), *Menstrual Bleeding and Pain Disorders from Adolescence to Menopause*, ISGE Series,
https://doi.org/10.1007/978-3-031-55300-4_12

have concerns about treatment-induced infertility, and in some cases these concerns influence their treatment decision [5–8]. However, the discussion about CIA and infertility risk between oncologists and their patients remains limited [5, 6].

CIA is not the only situation of menstrual absence: Obstetrician–gynecologists frequently are consulted either before the initiation of cancer treatment to request menstrual suppression or during an episode of severe heavy bleeding to stop bleeding emergently. Adolescents undergoing cancer treatment are at high risk of abnormal menstrual bleeding as a direct result of hematologic malignancies or as a secondary effect of chemotherapy, radiation therapy, or pretreatment regimens for stem cell or bone marrow transplantation, all of which may induce myelosuppression leading to thrombocytopenia. Additional considerations include the potential for disruption of the hypothalamic–pituitary–gonadal axis during cancer treatment leading to anovulatory bleeding.

In the following chapter, the most common menstrual disorders connected with anticancer treatment will be treated.

2　Chemotherapy-Induced Amenorrhea

The link between adjuvant chemotherapy and amenorrhea has been well established, but the specific effect of individual chemotherapeutic agents and regimens on risk for amenorrhea has not been well characterized. The most important drawback on the current literature is the lack of uniform definition of CIA. In the mid-1990s, a systematic review by Bines et al. underscored the need for uniform definition of CIA and proposed one based on the duration of amenorrhea (>6 months) [10]. A similar definition has been adopted from the American College of Obstetricians and Gynecologists based on the current systematic review and the evidence derived from studies with long-term follow-up, where resumption of menses occurs often within 2 years of CIA [11, 12]; Zavos and Valachis suggested that the definition of CIA should be based on the presence of amenorrhea for at least 2 years commencing within 2 years of chemotherapy with no resumption of menses during this period. One could argue that this definition is also problematic since there are some patients that resume menses even 2–3 years after CIA [9]; however, they assumed that the 2-year cutoff is an acceptable compromise between the necessity for a uniform and reliable definition and the resources that a prospective study investigating the risk for CIA in cancer patients is needed.

Irrespective of the definition used for CIA, cessation of menses is only a surrogate marker for ovarian function and should not be considered synonymous to true ovarian failure. In fact, it has been found that estrogen levels can remain high despite the presence of CIA for more than 12 months [9]. Conversely, recovery of menstruation after chemotherapy does not rule out follicular depletion, and fertility cannot be guaranteed [13]. These observations suggest that more accurate indicators of ovarian function are needed to properly inform cancer patients about their risk for infertility due to cancer treatment. Among several markers that have been studied, anti-Müllerian hormone (AMH) seems to be the most promising one. Indeed, serum AMH has been associated with recovery of ovarian function in young women during and after chemotherapy [14].

3   Etiologies and Pathogenesis

3.1   Gonadotoxicity of Anticancer Treatments

Cancer and anticancer treatments may affect post-treatment ovarian function by a reduction in ovarian reserve (i.e., the primordial follicle pool); a disturbed hormonal balance; or anatomical or functional changes to the ovaries, uterus, cervix, or vagina. Reduced ovarian function may result in infertility and premature ovarian insufficiency (POI): POI is defined as oligo-/amenorrhea for >4 months and follicle-stimulating hormone (FSH) levels of >25 IU/l on two occasions, 4 weeks apart, before the age of 40 years. Notably, in cancer patients, menstrual function can resume many months after completion of treatment; in addition, infertility and POI may occur despite temporary resumption of menses [3].

CIA is mainly due to damage to growing follicles that occurs within weeks after CIA initiation and is often transient. Depending on age, pretreatment ovarian reserve, and type of treatment, exhaustion of the primordial follicle pool may occur with subsequent POI. Because of their cell cycle nonspecific mode of action, alkylating agents induce the greatest damage, not only to growing follicles but also to oocytes, resulting in a striking reduction of the primordial follicle pool [15].

The impact of most targeted agents (including monoclonal antibodies and small molecules) and immunotherapy is largely unknown. Limited data for the anti-human epidermal growth factor receptor 2 (HER2) agents trastuzumab and/or lapatinib indicate no apparent gonadotoxicity [16]. An increased risk of ovarian dysfunction in patients treated with bevacizumab cannot be excluded [3]. Endocrine treatments may have an indirect effect on fertility by delaying time to pregnancy. A higher risk of treatment-related amenorrhea with the use of tamoxifen following chemotherapy has been described in several studies. Nonetheless, no impact on AMH levels has been shown [17, 18].

4   Prognostic Factors

Women who have had cancer are at an increased risk of early menopause and POI as a result of ovarian follicle depletion, stromal fibrosis, and vascular injury after chemotherapy and radiotherapy [19]. Early menopause has a negative effect on quality of life [20] and is associated with osteoporosis, cardiovascular disease, and psychosocial disorders such as depression. Even survivors in whom ovarian function resumes or is maintained after cancer treatment might face a shortened *window of fertility* [21]. The extent of the damage to the ovary depends on the type and dose of chemotherapy [3], the radiotherapy dose, fractionation scheme, and irradiation field [22] and the ovarian reserve before treatment (Table 1).

Table 1 Risks of treatment-related amenorrhea in female patients

Risks of treatment-related amenorrhea in female patients[a]		
Degree of risk	Treatment type/regimen	Comments
High risk (>80%)[b]	Hematopoietic stem cell transplantation (especially alkylating agent-based myeloablative conditioning with cyclophosphamide, busulfan, melphalan, or total body RT)	
	EBRT > 6 Gy to a field including the ovaries	
	6 cycles of CMF, CEF, CAF, or TAC in women of >40 years	Significant decline in AMH levels after treatment early menopause
	6e8 cycles of escalated BEACOPP in women of >30 years	Significant decline in AMH levels after treatment
Intermediate risk (20%–80%)[c]	6 cycles of CMF, CEF, CAF, or TAC in women of 30–39 years	Significant decline in AMH levels after treatment early menopause
	4 cycles of AC in women of >40 years	Significant decline in AMH levels after treatment
	4 cycles of AC/EC/taxane	Significant decline in AMH levels after treatment
	4 cycles of dd (F)EC/dd taxane	
	6e8 cycles of escalated BEACOPP in women of <30 years	Significant decline in AMH levels after treatment
	6 cycles of CHOP in women of >35 years	Early menopause
	6 cycles of DA-EPOCH in women of >35 years	Significant decline in AMH levels after treatment
	FOLFOX in women of >40 years	
Low risk (<20%)[d]	6 cycles of CMF, CEF, CAF, or TAC in women of <30 years	Significant decline in AMH levels after treatment early menopause
	4 cycles of AC in women of <40 years	Significant decline in AMH levels after treatment
	2 cycles of escalated BEACOPP	Significant decline in AMH levels after treatment

Table 1 (continued)

Risks of treatment-related amenorrhea in female patients[a]		
Degree of risk	Treatment type/regimen	Comments
	ABVD	Insignificant decline in AMH levels after treatment
	6 cycles of CHOP in women of <35 years	Early menopause
	6 cycles of DA-EPOCH in women of <35 years	Significant decline in AMH levels after treatment
	AML therapy (anthracycline/cytarabine)	Insignificant decline in AMH levels after treatment
	ALL therapy (multi-agent)	Insignificant decline in AMH levels after treatment
	Multi-agent ChT for osteosarcoma (doxorubicin, cisplatin, methotrexate, ifosfamide) in women of <35 years	
	Multi-agent ChT for Ewing's sarcoma (doxorubicin, vincristine, dactinomycin, cyclophosphamide, ifosfamide, etoposide) in women of <35 years	
	FOLFOX in women of >40 years	
	Antimetabolites and vinca alkaloids	
	BEP or EP in women of <30 years	
	Radioactive iodine (I-131)	Decline in AMH levels after treatment
	Bevacizumab	
Unknown risk	Platinum- and taxane-based ChT	
	Most targeted therapies (including monoclonal antibodies and small molecules)	
	Immunotherapy	

ABVD doxorubicin, bleomycin, vinblastine, dacarbazine, *AC* doxorubicin, cyclophosphamide, *ALL* acute lymphoid leukemia, *AMH* anti-Müllerian hormone, *AML* acute myeloid leukemia, *BEACOPP* bleomycin, etoposide, doxorubicin, cyclophosphamide, vincristine, prednisone, procarbazine, *BEP* bleomycin, etoposide, cisplatin, *CAF* cyclophosphamide, doxorubicin, 5-fluorouracil, *CEF* cyclophosphamide, epirubicin, 5-fluorouracil, *CHOP* cyclophosphamide, doxorubicin, vincristine, prednisone, *ChT* chemotherapy, *CMF* cyclo-phosphamide, methotrexate, 5-fluorouracil, *DA-EPOCH* dose-adjusted etoposide, prednisone, vincristine, cyclophosphamide, doxorubicin, *dd* dose dense, *EBRT* external beam radiotherapy, *EC* epirubicin, cyclophosphamide, *EP* etoposide, cisplatin, *F* fluorouracil, *FOLFOX* folinic acid, 5-fluorouracil, oxaliplatin, *Gy* Gray, *RT* radiotherapy, *TAC* docetaxel, doxorubicin, cyclophosphamide
[a]Adapted from [3]
[b] >80% risk of permanent amenorrhea
[c] >40–60% risk of permanent amenorrhea
[d]<20% risk of permanent amenorrhea

Regarding the risk factors for CIA, age is the strongest risk factor (sixfold increased risk for CIA for patients <40 years old), whereas tamoxifen use is associated with nearly twofold increased risk for CIA. On the contrary, age at menarche and BMI do not influence the risk for CIA. These observations are supported by a high level of evidence [9]. Age is an important marker of ovarian reserve, as are the serum markers estradiol, inhibin B, follicle-stimulating hormone, and AMH. AMH has emerged as an especially strong predictor of ovarian function after chemotherapy. A rapid and substantial reduction of circulating AMH concentration is noted in adults after the start of chemotherapy [23], and recent data suggest that AMH concentrations before the start of chemotherapy, and the reduction and recovery of AMH during and after chemotherapy, might predict the amount of ovarian damage [24]. These data suggest a crucial role for AMH in the identification of patients who might benefit from fertility preservation and which approach will optimize future fecundity. However, in prepubertal and peripubertal girls, AMH concentrations should be interpreted with caution because they cannot unequivocally predict reproductive lifespan [21]. Long-term follow-up data for AMH concentrations decades after cancer treatment are not yet available to establish the predictive potential of AMH with regard to reproductive lifespan in cancer survivors.

Follicle depletion is the hallmark of ovarian damage and is most pronounced in women given alkylating agents, such as cyclophosphamide [24], and in those who receive total-body irradiation before hematopoietic stem cell transplantation or direct irradiation of the ovaries. The precise mechanism by which cyclophosphamide affects the primordial follicle pool is not entirely understood, but recent studies investigating the effect of cyclophosphamide in mouse ovaries suggest that cyclophosphamide results in activation rather than apoptosis of primordial follicles [25], via upregulation of the PI3K/PTEN/Akt signalling pathway. According to these data, cyclophosphamide causes apoptosis of larger growing follicles, with cyclophosphamide-induced primordial follicle activation ultimately resulting in follicle burnout.

Other chemotherapeutic drugs might directly damage the growing oocyte or the highly proliferative granulosa cells within the developing follicle. These drugs might also cause follicle depletion indirectly, by damaging growing follicles and enhancing recruitment of primordial follicles to deplete the follicle pool or by altering the ovarian stroma [19]. An understanding of the gonadotoxic mechanisms of chemotherapy is needed to design effective agents that protect against iatrogenic depletion of ovarian follicles in young patients with cancer.

Taking into account the effect of fertility issues on patients' quality of life, the American Society of Clinical Oncology recommends that oncologists discuss the risk of infertility and fertility preservation options in patients with cancer as early as possible before treatment starts [9].

5   Chemotherapy-Induced Ovarian Failure

Chemotherapy-associated ovarian failure (COF) refers to disruption of both endocrine and reproductive ovarian function, after exposure to chemotherapy. It is defined as either the absence of regular menses in premenopausal female patients or as increased FSH levels (>40 IU/L) [26].

In 2006, the American Association of Clinical Oncology attempted to sort antineoplastic regimens, according to the associated fertility compromise risk. Hematopoietic stem cell transplant (HSCT) initiation regimens steadily compromise patients' fertility, while gonadotoxicity of adjuvant chemotherapy regimens against early breast cancer varies with duration of exposure and patient's age. Characteristically, triple agent combinations, such as CMF (cyclophosphamide, methotrexate, fluorouracil), entail a high risk of infertility if administered for more than four cycles in women older than 40, whereas the risk is significantly reduced for younger patients. Notably, vincristine, methotrexate, and fluorouracil do not impose considerable fertility hazards, while there are no sufficient data regarding taxanes, oxaliplatin, and targeted treatments [27].

Considering the finite number of follicles available in the ovaries and their coexistence in different stages of development, variable pathophysiologic mechanisms have been proposed to underlie chemotherapy-induced ovarian failure. These include:

- "Accelerated" ovarian follicle maturation: Chemotherapy agents induce apoptosis of mature, functioning ovarian follicles, resulting in depression of estrogen and anti-Müllerian hormone negative feedback on the gonadotropic cells of the anterior pituitary. Persistently elevated gonadotropins may accelerate maturation of premature ovarian follicles, which, in their turn, enter apoptosis under systematic chemotherapy, thus the gradual exhaustion of ovarian follicle deposit [26, 28]. Supporting evidence comes from histologic studies of murine ovarian tissue, in cyclophosphamide-treated mice, showing increased population of early growing follicles, in parallel with elimination of the quiescent ones. The enhanced phosphorylation of proteins involved in the maturation of primordial follicles seems to be mediated via the PI3K/PTEN/Akt signaling pathway, which may also be activated due to a direct effect of chemotherapy on oocytes and on pregranulosa cells supporting them [25].
- Direct quiescent follicle DNA damage: Non-cell cycle specific chemotherapeutics, such as alkylating agents and doxorubicin, can induce formation of crosslinks in the DNA of non-dividing, dormant oocytes. The subsequent accumulation of DNA strand breaks activates the pro-apoptotic intracellular pathways, leading to apoptosis of the affected ovarian follicles [29]. Relevant supporting evidence derives from studies of human oocyte in vitro cultures and human ovarian xenograft murine models, exposed to doxorubicin and cyclophosphamide, revealing double strand breaks and features of apoptotic death in premature oocytes [27].

– Disrupted ovarian vascularization: Chemotherapy may compromise the functionality of ovarian vasculature and stroma supporting the gonadal cells. Local vascular spasm reducing ovarian blood flow, fibrosis of the ovarian cortex affecting blood vessel formation, and inhibition of angiogenesis are some of the described associated mechanisms. Relative evidence has been found in in vitro and murine xenograft studies of human ovarian tissue, as well as mouse ovaries, exposed to doxorubicin [27, 29].

6 Risk of CIA in Patients with Breast Cancer

The incidence of breast cancer in young women has been relatively stable around the world during the last 20 years. However, breast cancer in young women remains a challenge for the oncologist: the high risk for recurrence in this patient population has led to more aggressive therapeutic strategies including adjuvant chemotherapy that improves the survival rates, but, at the same time, chemotherapy negatively influences patients' quality of life.

As explained before, the rate of CIA was increased by age and adjuvant chemotherapy regimen, as reported in Table 1. A flowchart to illustrate the risk classification of CIA based on age and type of chemotherapy is shown on Fig. 1.

This flowchart could serve as a helpful guide for oncologists during the discussion with their patients on fertility issues before decisions on adjuvant therapy are made. The discussion should include the inherent risk for amenorrhea of each

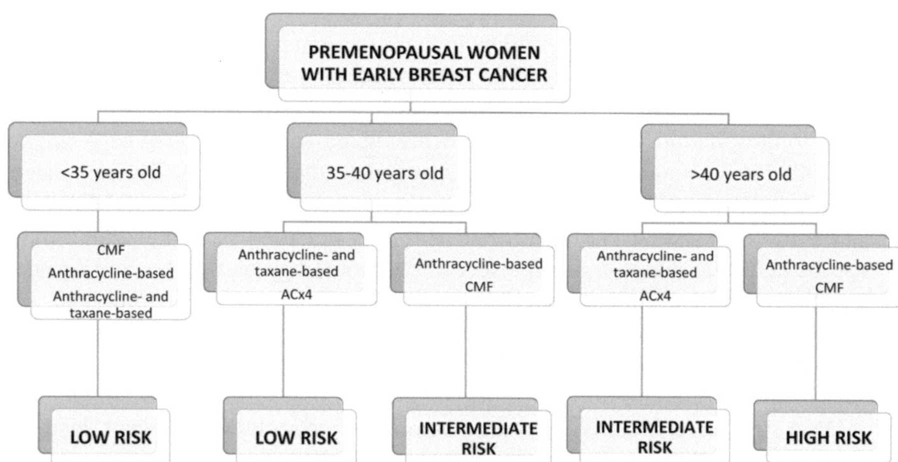

Fig. 1 Flowchart of risk for chemotherapy-induced amenorrhea based on age and type of chemotherapy. *AC* doxorubicin-cyclophosphamide, *CMF* cyclophosphamide-methotrexate-fluorouracil. (Adapted from [9])

chemotherapy combination, the potential role of risk factors (including age, tamoxifen use) on this risk, the fertility preservation options, and the psychosocial aspects of the decision [9].

7   Radiotherapy-Induced Ovarian Failure

Radiotherapy (RT) exposure causes a reduction in the number of ovarian follicles and has an adverse effect on uterine and endometrial function; the gonadotoxic effect of RT is dependent on the RT field, dose, and fractionation schedule, with single doses more toxic than multiple fractions [3]. RT-related ovarian follicle loss already occurs at doses higher than 2 Gy. The effective sterilizing dose at which 97.5% of patients are expected to develop immediate POI decreases with increasing age at the time of treatment, ranging from 16 Gy at 20 years to 14 Gy at 30 years. RT also induces loss of uterine elasticity in a dose-dependent manner. This interferes with uterine distension, with increased risk throughout pregnancy [30]. A potential negative impact of cancer on ovarian reserve has been described for young women with lymphoma but not for patients with other malignancies.

7.1   *Predicting Age of Ovarian Failure After Radiation*

As survival rates for children and adolescents treated for cancer continue to improve, a population of young women of reproductive age emerges for whom issues of fertile potential are paramount. Impaired fecundity and premature ovarian failure are recognized potential late sequelae of radiotherapy to the ovaries [22].

The human ovary contains a fixed pool of primordial oocytes, maximal at 5 months of gestational age, which declines with increasing age in a biexponential fashion, culminating in the menopause at an average age of 50–51 years. For any given age, the size of the oocyte pool can be estimated based on a mathematical model of decline [22, 31]. The rate of oocyte decline represents an instantaneous rate of temporal change determined by the remaining population pool, which increases around age 37 years when approximately 25,000 primordial oocytes remain and precedes the menopause by 12–14 years [32]. Reproductive aging in women is due to ovarian oocyte depletion with approximately 1000 oocytes remaining at the menopause. Assessment of ovarian reserve and reproductive age in healthy women remains a challenge.

Radiotherapy may be used either alone or in combination with surgery and chemotherapy to provide local disease control for solid tumors. Because of its established late sequelae on immature and developing tissues, irradiation is used cautiously, especially in children and adolescents. Total body, craniospinal axis, whole abdominal, or pelvic irradiation potentially expose the ovaries to irradiation and may cause premature ovarian failure. The degree of impairment is related to the volume treated, total radiation dose, fractionation schedule, and age at the time of treatment [31, 33]. The number of primordial oocytes present at the time of treatment, together with the biologic dose of radiotherapy received by the ovaries, will determine the fertile "window" and influence the age at premature ovarian failure. Assessing the extent of radiation-induced damage of the primordial oocytes and predicting the impact on fertile potential has been challenging. An understanding of ovarian follicle dynamics has allowed us to determine the radiosensitivity of the human oocyte to be 2 Gy [33]. Application of this estimate has made it possible to determine the surviving fraction of the primordial oocyte pool for a given dose of radiotherapy and therefore predict the age (with confidence intervals) of premature ovarian failure by applying a mathematical model of decay.

Radiotherapy is frequently used in combination with chemotherapy for the treatment of cancer. Potentially gonadotoxic chemotherapy may be a contributory factor to the development of a premature menopause. However, when the dose of radiotherapy received by the ovaries is at, or approaching, the effective sterilizing dose, the additional contribution of chemotherapy is likely to be minimal. For smaller doses of radiation to the ovary, such as for spinal irradiation, the contribution of chemotherapy will play a more significant role. Several agents have been described to cause ovarian damage, including procarbazine, chlorambucil, and cyclophosphamide with the extent of the damage dependent on the agent administered and dose received [22]. As with radiotherapy, progressively smaller doses are required to produce ovarian failure with increasing age, reflecting the natural decline in the oocyte pool. Although the mechanism of cytotoxic chemotherapy-induced damage to the ovary is uncertain, exhaustion of the oocyte pool is likely.

A successful term pregnancy will depend on a normally functioning hypothalamic–pituitary–ovarian axis and a uterine environment that is not only receptive to implantation but also able to accommodate normal growth of the fetus. The degree of damage to the uterus depends on the total radiation dose and the site of irradiation. The prepubertal uterus is more vulnerable to the effects of pelvic irradiation with doses of radiation between 14 and 30 Gy likely to result in uterine dysfunction. High-dose pelvic radiotherapy in young women will have long-term effects on the uterine vasculature and development.

When counseling patients after treatment with smaller doses of radiotherapy, around 3 Gy, which can be associated with radiotherapy to the craniospinal axis, the physicians can be relatively optimistic and reassuring that they will have a significant reproductive window before premature ovarian failure occurs. The fertile window will be attenuated with increasing doses of radiotherapy. For girls who are likely to be rendered sterile before the onset of menarche, it will enable physicians to realistically counsel their patients and families when discussing options for preservation of ovarian function at the time of diagnosis before treatment has commenced. A number of strategies to protect the ovaries and preserve fertility during cancer therapy have been attempted [21, 34]. Limitation of radiation dose to the ovary is sometimes practiced in adult women, but in children is technically difficult.

8   Prophylactic Menstrual Suppression

CIA is not the only situation of menstrual absence: Obstetrician–gynecologists frequently are consulted either before the initiation of cancer treatment to request menstrual suppression or during an episode of severe heavy bleeding to stop bleeding emergently.

Adolescents undergoing cancer treatment are at high risk of abnormal menstrual bleeding as a direct result of hematologic malignancies or as a secondary effect of chemotherapy, radiation therapy, or pretreatment regimens for stem cell or bone marrow transplantation, all of which may induce myelosuppression leading to thrombocytopenia. Additional considerations include the potential for disruption of the hypothalamic–pituitary–gonadal axis during cancer treatment leading to anovulatory bleeding. Also, even normal menstrual blood loss may pose a threat to adolescents who already are anemic, thrombocytopenic, or both, from hematologic malignancies or cancer treatments. Thus, obstetrician–gynecologists frequently are consulted either before the initiation of cancer treatment to request menstrual suppression or during an episode of severe heavy bleeding to stop bleeding emergently [35]. Therapy for both menstrual suppression and management of acute bleeding episodes should be tailored to the patient, the cancer diagnosis and treatment plan, and the individual's contraceptive needs. Because of the complex nature of cancer care, collaboration with the adolescent's oncologist is highly recommended. Options for menstrual suppression include gonadotropin-releasing hormone agonist (GnRHa), progestin-only therapy, and combined hormonal contraception [36]. Adolescents presenting emergently with severe uterine bleeding usually require only medical management; surgical management rarely is required. Considerations when choosing an appropriate treatment for acute bleeding include the patient's current menstrual status, current hemoglobin and platelet count, expected nadirs, planned cancer treatments, risk of thromboembolism, and request for contraception. If a patient is treated with leuprolide acetate for menstrual suppression, this should not be considered a contraceptive method because ovulation may not be universally suppressed [37].

An American College of Obstetricians and Gynecologists' Committee on Adolescent Health Care has been updated to make treatment recommendations based on more recent studies, to address specific concerns about the use of combined hormonal contraception (CHC) in cancer patients, and to update nonmedical management to include the intrauterine Foley balloon.

8.1 Menstrual Suppression

8.1.1 Gonadotropin-Releasing Hormone Agonists

Gonadotropin-releasing hormone agonists are highly effective at inducing menstrual suppression when initiated before cancer treatment [36]. The primary role of GnRHA is for menstrual suppression. Though they appear to have a protective effect on the ovary during chemotherapy in terms of resumption of menstruation and treatment-related premature ovarian failure, there is no conclusive evidence demonstrating efficacy of GnRHa in fertility preservation [37].

Most of the data on GnRHa focuses on the use of leuprolide acetate, a synthetic GnRHa that acts as a potent inhibitor of gonadotropin release when given in therapeutic doses. Studies, including a systematic review of women undergoing cancer treatment, report high rates of amenorrhea with leuprolide acetate (ranging from 73% to 96%) [38].

After an initial flare response that causes a transient increase in circulating gonadotropins and sex steroids, leuprolide acetate reliably causes a hypoestrogenic state in 2 weeks. Therefore, bleeding may occur for 2–3 weeks after the first injection until hormone levels decrease and endometrial proliferation ceases. When initiating treatment with leuprolide, adding norethindrone acetate 5 mg daily will help mitigate breakthrough bleeding and other adverse effects of leuprolide. It may be given in doses of 3.75 mg intramuscularly monthly or 11.5 mg intramuscularly every 12 weeks. The 12-week formulation decreases the risk of more frequent monthly injections that may be due at a time of treatment-induced thrombocytopenia. If intramuscular injections are contraindicated, subcutaneous formulations are available [37].

Disadvantages of leuprolide acetate include the expected adverse effects related to a low-estrogen state, such as vasomotor symptoms and bone density loss. When leuprolide acetate is used to treat endometriosis in adolescents, add-back therapy with a progestin (such as norethindrone acetate 5 mg once daily) has been shown to preserve bone mass and substantially reduce vasomotor symptoms without increasing the rate of bleeding. Treatment should be individualized; certain cancer patients, depending on potential risks and benefits, may be candidates for combined add-back therapy.

8.1.2 Progestin-Only Therapy

Daily administration of oral progestins allows for decreased endometrial proliferation and prevention of menses. Options for progestin-only oral therapies are medroxyprogesterone acetate (10–20 mg/day), norethindrone acetate (5–15 mg/day), drospirenone (4 mg/day), and norethindrone (0.35 mg/day). Drospirenone (4 mg/day) and norethindrone (0.35 mg/day) also provide contraception but do not confer the same degree of amenorrhea as other oral progestins, and unscheduled bleeding is relatively common in users [38, 39].

Use of depot medroxyprogesterone acetate (DMPA) results in relatively high rates of amenorrhea over time, with rates at 12–24 months reaching approximately 50–70% in the general population [40]. However, initial irregular bleeding with DMPA makes it a less reliable method for rapid therapeutic menstrual suppression, and episodes of breakthrough bleeding can be challenging to manage, particularly in patients who are not candidates for adjuvant estrogen. It is classified as a Category 2 method (the advantages of using the method generally outweigh the theoretical or proven risks) among those with a history of VTE and active cancer according to the Centers for Disease Control and Prevention's US Medical Eligibility Criteria for Contraceptive Use. Data on the use of progestin-only methods by patients with cancer are limited. Depot medroxyprogesterone acetate typically is administered every 12 weeks, but the dosing interval can be shortened to achieve amenorrhea quickly. Its long dosing interval of up to 3 months minimizes concerns over adherence and is a good option for patients unable to swallow or tolerate pills. A subcutaneous formulation (dose of 104 mg) is available and is recommended for adolescents with thrombocytopenia who are at risk of developing an intramuscular hematoma with intramuscular administration [37].

Although there are limited data regarding menstrual management with an LNG-IUD in patients undergoing cancer treatment, it is a reasonable option to manage heavy menstrual bleeding in a patient with benign or malignant disease. Furthermore, the World Health Organization and the Centers for Disease Control and Prevention state that IUDs can be used safely in women with immunosuppression because of cancer treatment. Although initial irregular bleeding may limit its use, many studies in noncancer patients have demonstrated the superiority of the 52 micrograms LNG-IUD over oral medroxyprogesterone acetate, norethindrone acetate, DMPA, and CHC for long-term menstrual control [37].

If an adolescent had an LNG-IUD or the etonogestrel single-rod implant inserted before her cancer diagnosis and has infrequent bleeding or amenorrhea, it is reasonable to continue the method for menstrual suppression. However, if an adolescent had an implant inserted before her cancer diagnosis and experiences bothersome bleeding, the bleeding can be temporized with a norethindrone acetate or medroxyprogesterone taper and the implant continued.

8.1.3   Combined Hormonal Contraceptives

When used continuously, CHCs are effective for producing amenorrhea, although complete amenorrhea cannot be guaranteed. The Centers for Disease Control and Prevention's 2016 US Medical Eligibility Criteria for Contraceptive Use notes that when oral contraceptives primarily are used as therapy, rather than to prevent pregnancy, even in women where contraceptive use might be cautioned against or contraindicated (such as in those with cancer), the benefits from therapeutic use might outweigh the risks [37].

The decision to use estrogen in patients with cancer should be tailored to the individual patient after collaborative consideration of the risk–benefit ratio with the patient and the healthcare team; the patient should be closely monitored for known adverse effects such as liver toxicity and VTE.

8.1.4 Emergent Treatment of Acute Uterine Bleeding

Some adolescents may present with life-threatening bleeding in the setting of a new cancer diagnosis, whereas others who are undergoing myelosuppressive treatment may not have the time to benefit from prophylactic menstrual suppression and need more urgent therapy once bleeding occurs. Medical management is the initial approach for patients who are experiencing an episode of acute heavy bleeding. Surgical management should be considered for patients who are not clinically stable or for those whose conditions are not suitable for medical management or have failed to respond appropriately to medical management [41]. Some hormonal therapies that are used for menstrual suppression, such as leuprolide acetate, DMPA, LNG-IUD, and the etonogestrel implant, are not appropriate for the initial management of acute heavy bleeding because the onset of action is delayed, and, in some cases, the bleeding pattern is unpredictable. Instead, these therapies may be used in conjunction with therapy for acute bleeding to prevent future episodes of acute uterine bleeding. Ultrasonography can be useful to guide management. Endometrial thickness can guide whether the patient may benefit from progestin or estrogen.

9 Fertility Preservation Strategies

The assessment of fertility risk and the selection of an individualized strategy to optimize fecundity after cancer treatment are huge challenges and require intense cooperation between fertility preservation specialists, oncologists, other healthcare workers, and the patient. Guidelines developed on the basis of systematic reviews and scientific literature analyses recommend fertility preservation approaches by patient age, cancer type, type of treatment, presence of a male partner or patient preference for the use of banked donor sperm, time available for fertility preservation intervention, and the likelihood of ovarian metastasis. Established fertility preservation methods include oocyte and embryo cryopreservation, both derived from routine reproductive clinical practice, and ovarian transposition (oophoropexy), which can be offered to women undergoing pelvic irradiation [21] (Fig. 2).

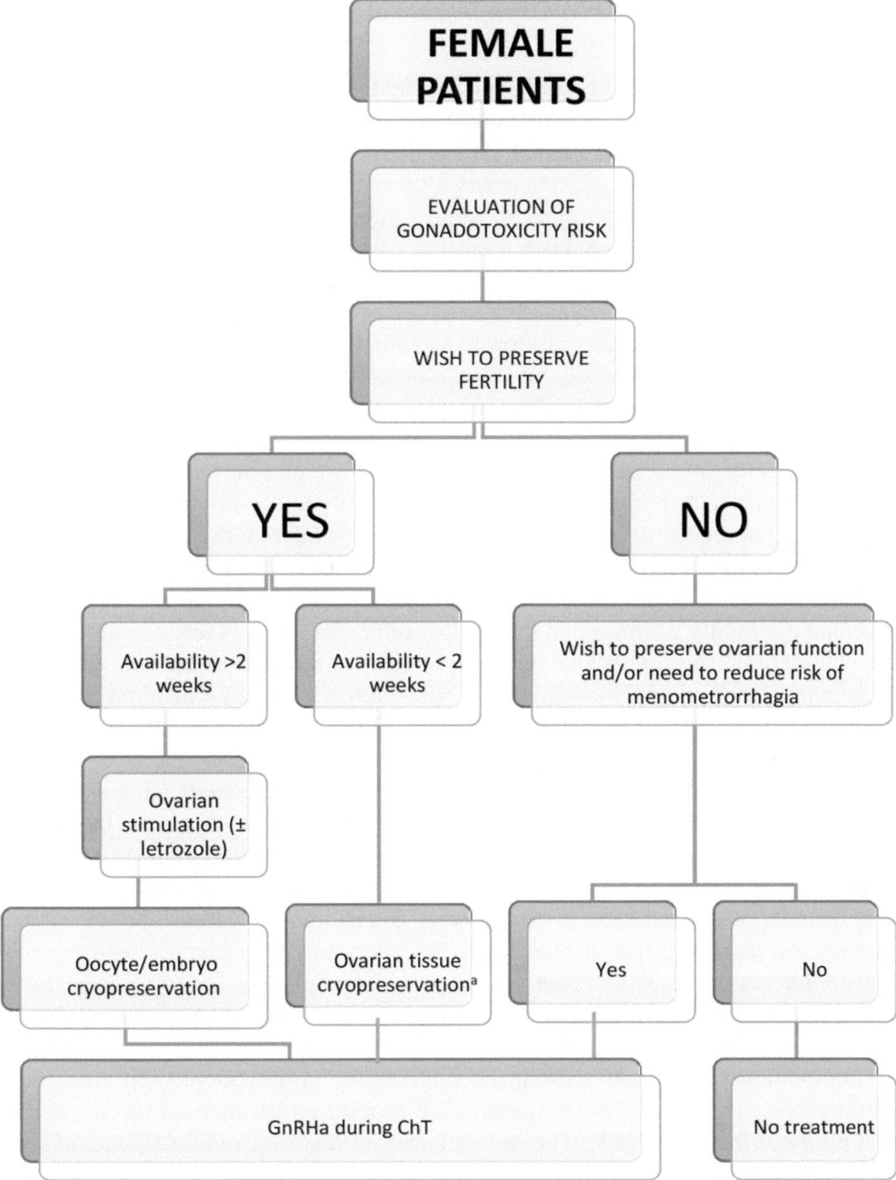

Fig. 2 Management flowchart for ovarian function and/or fertility preservation in female patients. *ChT* chemotherapy, *GnRHa* gonadotropin-releasing hormone agonist. [a]To be offered preferably in women 36 years of age and to be considered with particular caution in cases of acute leukemia or any solid tumor or hematological disease with pelvic involvement. (Adapted from [21])

9.1　Oocyte and Embryo Cryopreservation

Oocytes and embryos can be safely and efficiently cryopreserved before the initiation of anticancer treatments. While embryo cryopreservation is an established and reproducible technology, it requires the use of sperm and the presence of a partner or donor. Conversely, oocyte cryopreservation can be carried out without a partner, and so it is the preferred option for most post-pubertal women. The ability to cryopreserve oocytes has become much more successful in recent years since the development of ultra-rapid freezing (vitrification).

For oocyte and embryo cryopreservation, about 2 weeks of ovarian stimulation with gonadotropins is required, followed by follicle aspiration. Ovarian stimulation can be started at any time of the menstrual cycle ("random start stimulation"). Developments in ovarian stimulation protocols allow more rapid completion of the process than previously, without affecting their efficacy. However, timing is a crucial factor as the procedure must be completed before initiation of any chemotherapy. In women with a low ovarian reserve and without an urgent need to initiate anticancer treatments, double stimulation can be considered; this requires 4 weeks of treatment and approximately doubles the number of oocytes retrieved [3, 42].

The efficacy of oocyte and embryo cryopreservation to generate a subsequent pregnancy is tightly connected to the number of mature oocytes retrieved after ovarian stimulation. The number of retrieved oocytes is reduced in women with poor ovarian reserve (low AMH level due to ovarian surgery or age). The number of collected oocytes is age dependent, varying from 15.4–8.8 in women <26 years of age to 9.9–8.0 in women 36–40 years of age.

Ovarian stimulation can lead to side effects caused by the medication as well as complications during the oocyte pick-up, including bleeding from the ovary and pelvic infection. Severe ovarian hyperstimulation syndrome and clinically relevant bleeding or inflammation/infections after follicular aspiration in women with normal hematopoiesis are rare in the general infertility population and in cancer patients. An increased risk of bleeding or infection may be present in women with impaired hematopoiesis (i.e., neutropenic or with low platelet count), such as those with some hematological malignancies, and should be taken into account [3]. In estrogen-sensitive tumors, reduction of estradiol concentration is recommended during ovarian stimulation and can be achieved by co-treatment with aromatase inhibitors (e.g., letrozole 2×2.5 mg/day), which reduces estrogen serum concentration by more than 50% [43]. The use of letrozole does not reduce the number of mature oocytes obtained or their fertilization capacity; in addition, no effect on congenital abnormality rates in children has been observed.

Oocyte or embryo cryopreservation is indicated for women preferably <40 years of age who will be exposed to gonadotoxic anticancer therapies and who want to preserve their fertility. It is not indicated in women with serious coagulation defects or high risk of infections. Trans-abdominal monitoring and oocyte recovery may be possible in those for whom vaginal procedures are not possible or acceptable. Women choosing to store embryos created with their partner's sperm should be advised that the embryos will be the joint property of the couple; in the event of the relationship not continuing, there may be issues in using the embryos. An established collaboration between oncology and fertility units is crucial.

There is a need for data on all aspects of oocyte cryopreservation from larger series of women to clarify whether certain diagnoses may benefit from particular stimulation protocols, the effects on oocyte quality, and, most importantly, cumulative live birth rates. Future studies are also needed to investigate the benefits of combining different fertility preservation methods to increase pregnancy rates.

9.2 Ovarian Tissue Cryopreservation

Ovarian tissue cryopreservation is an alternative approach for preserving fertility before gonadotoxic treatments. While it is still regarded as experimental in some countries, the American Society for Reproductive Medicine suggests that it should be considered as an established procedure to be offered to carefully selected patients [3, 44].

Biopsies of the ovarian cortex or unilateral ovariectomy are usually carried out by laparoscopy under general anesthesia. Although vitrification is quicker and less expensive, slow freezing remains the standard of care because almost all pregnancies achieved after transplantation have been obtained using this procedure. Ovarian tissue cryopreservation should be offered only in laboratories with specific expertise and facilities to support safe tissue cryopreservation and storage for subsequent autologous transplantation, with necessary regulation. The "hub and spoke" model, with ovarian surgery carried out locally and tissue transported to a central laboratory, may be preferred.

Transplantation, either orthotopic or heterotopic, is currently the only method available in clinical practice to restore ovarian function and fertility using cryopreserved ovarian tissue. As with oocyte and embryo cryopreservation, the main factor affecting success rate is age: women of younger age at ovarian tissue cryopreservation have better fertility outcomes after ovarian tissue transplantation than older women, with only a few pregnancies achieved in women over 36 years of age [45].

Ovarian tissue collection and transplantation are usually carried out by laparoscopy. Surgical risk is considered low, and complications (e.g., conversion laparotomy, bleeding, reintervention for cutaneous infection, bladder lesion, or minor complications) are rare (0.2–1.4%) [46]. The procedure should not be proposed to patients with high surgical/anesthesia risks related to their disease and ideally should be done at the same time as other procedures that require anesthesia. The risk of disease transmission during transplantation due to residual neoplastic cells within the ovarian cortex is one of the major safety concerns, especially in pelvic cancers or systemic diseases such as leukemia. Several diseases at advanced stages, such as Burkitt's lymphoma, non-Hodgkin's lymphoma, breast cancer, and sarcoma, might also carry a risk of ovarian involvement. Nevertheless, ovarian tissue should always be carefully analyzed before grafting using all available technologies, such as immunohistochemistry and molecular markers, according to the disease. Xenografting has also been used in this context. Data on children are reassuring as no congenital malformations have been reported [3].

Ovarian tissue cryopreservation is appropriate when the time available before starting anticancer treatments is too short for ovarian stimulation and oocyte or embryo cryopreservation. Although there is no clear consensus on the maximum age for ovarian tissue cryopreservation, it is usually recommended to offer this procedure only to women <36 years of age [3, 45]. Ovarian tissue cryopreservation can also be carried out after an initial, low-intensity gonadotoxic treatment regimen in order to reduce the risk of neoplastic cells being present in the ovary (i.e., in leukemia patients) or when the patient's initial health condition contraindicates an immediate procedure.

Research is ongoing to improve tissue function after grafting using several tools, including human adipose tissue-derived stem cells, mesenchymal stem cells, and decellularized scaffolds.

9.3 *Ovarian Transposition and Gonadal Shielding During RT*

Two options exist for protecting ovaries from RT: trans- position of the ovaries before RT and gonadal shielding during RT.

Ovarian transposition outside the planned RT field is a routinely used technique to minimize ovarian follicle RT exposure. Although both laparotomic and laparoscopic approaches are possible, the procedure is mostly carried out by laparoscopy to accelerate recovery and avoid postponing RT [3]. The ovary is mobilized with its vascular pedicle, and the location is marked with radio-opaque clips to allow identification of the transposed ovary. It is possible to transpose only one ovary, but better results are achieved with a bilateral procedure. Transposition of the ovary into subcutaneous tissue is another option, but it is associated with a higher risk of cyst formation [47]. Transposed ovaries can be safely punctured for oocyte retrieval. In certain cases, ovaries can be returned to their original location after RT. The rate of retained ovarian function is approximately 65% in patients undergoing surgery and RT [48]. Reasons for failure include necrosis related to vascular impairment and migration after insufficient fixation. Success rate is influenced by the method of evaluation (presence of menstrual cycle, FSH levels, AMH levels) and the duration of follow-up (as ovarian function decreases over time). The surgical risk of ovarian transposition is similar to other gynecological procedures (i.e., risk of bowel and vessel injury). Risk of developing ovarian carcinoma in a transposed ovary is extremely low. This could be reduced even further when the fallopian tubes are resected during the surgical procedure [48].

Gonadal shielding during RT by lead blocks reduces the expected RT dose to 4–5 Gy [3]. The minimum free margin should be 2 cm in order to reduce the risk of gonadal irradiation due to inner organ movement. Ovarian transposition and gonadal shielding are indicated in women <40 years of age who are scheduled to receive pelvic RT for cervical (if there is a low risk of ovarian metastasis or recurrence), vaginal, rectal, or anal cancers, Hodgkin's or non-Hodgkin's lymphoma in the pelvis, or Ewing's sarcoma of the pelvis. Long-term follow-up evaluating the risks of transposition and fertility rates after RT completion is needed.

9.4 Need to Reduce Gonadotoxicity: Medical Gonadoprotection

There has been extraordinary interest in medical agents that can potentially preserve fertility from the ovarian toxicity of chemotherapy. In this sense, temporary ovarian suppression obtained by administering a GnRHa has been studied as a strategy to reduce the gonadotoxic effect of chemotherapy [49]. When ovarian suppression with GnRHa is offered, GnRHa should be started at least 1 week before the initiation of systemic gonadotoxic treatment and prolonged until after the administration of the last chemotherapy cycle [50]. The debate on the efficacy of GnRHa for fertility preservation is still heated, but the 2018 ASCO guidelines recommended that GnRHa may be offered to premenopausal patients for reducing the likelihood of chemotherapy-induced ovarian insufficiency [51]. Nowadays, studies regarding the role of GnRHa as a fertility preservation treatment are evolving. In fact, the difference in the efficacy of GnRHa could not be assigned to the type of cancer, but rather to the regimen of chemotherapy. It is well known that gonadotoxic impact depends on the type of chemotherapeutic agent and the duration of administration [52]. The most common chemotherapy regimen used for the treatment of gynecological cancers (epithelial ovarian cancer) includes a combination of a platinum agent (carboplatin) and a taxane (paclitaxel). Currently, there is a lack of robust evidence to advise and recommend women on the risk of gonadotoxicity associated with this combination. Bleomycin, etoposide, and cisplatin (BEP) or etoposide and cisplatin (EP) chemotherapy regimens are often used for the treatment of non-epithelial ovarian cancers. Overall, chemotherapy regimens used for young women with gynecological cancers are considered to be associated with a low risk of gonadotoxicity, but this risk seems to be different according to the type of chemotherapy agent, the dose and length of exposure, and the age of the patient [3]. To investigate the impact of newer gonadotoxic treatments (including targeted agents and immunotherapy) on ovarian function, ovarian reserve and fertility potential of cancer patients should be considered a research priority. Instead, the gonadotoxic effect of chemotherapy in premenopausal women with early breast cancer is well known; the highest risk of gonadotoxicity is associated with the administration of the alkylating agent cyclophosphamide, commonly given as part of (neo) adjuvant chemotherapy regimens [53].

After more than 30 years of research and controversy in the gonadotoxicity battles, five theoretical mechanisms could explain how the GnRHa could minimize the gonadotoxic effect of chemotherapy:

1. Simulating the prepubertal hormonal milieu: GnRHa treatment has been identified to induce an initial release of gonadotropins, which desensitize the GnRH receptors on the pituitary gonadotropes, preventing pulsatile GnRH secretion, thus resulting in a hypogonadotropic, prepubertal hormonal milieu. In this prepubertal hypogonadotropic milieu, the follicles remain in the quiescent phase and are less vulnerable to chemotherapy-induced gonadotoxicity. Therefore, the administration of GnRHa, after the initial flare-up effect, decreases FSH concentration through pituitary desensitization, preventing the secretion of growth factors by the more advanced FSH-dependent follicles and secondarily preserving more primordial follicles (PMFs), which are metabolically inactive, in the dormant stage.

2. Interrupting the burnout effect: the administration of GnRHa may interfere with the accelerated follicle recruitment induced by chemotherapy by desensitizing the GnRH receptors in the pituitary gland, preventing an increase of FSH level despite low estrogen and inhibin concentrations.

3. Decreased utero-ovarian perfusion: a result of the hypoestrogenic milieu generated by pituitary-gonadal desensitization. The decreased utero-ovarian perfusion could result in a reduction of exposure of the ovaries to injuries caused by chemotherapeutic agents.

4. A possible direct effect mediated by ovarian GnRH receptors: human gonads also contain GnRH receptors and the activation of the ovarian GnRH receptor may decrease apoptosis.

5. Possible protection of ovarian germinative stem cells (GSCs): in patients undergoing chemotherapy, high menopausal FSH levels and undetectable AMH levels have been observed. Approximately a year after the chemotherapeutic ovarian insult, FSH concentrations have been shown to decrease to normal levels, and AMH has been found to increase in a large number of patients co-treated with GnRHa. Based on these clinical findings, it has been speculated that the administration of GnRHa may interact with these protected GSCs through some pathways essential for the initiation of folliculogenesis, maturation, and secretion of AMH, inhibin, and estrogens; and the latter two lead to a decrease in FSH levels to normal [54].

For premenopausal women interested in fertility preservation, with the hope of reducing chemotherapy-induced ovarian insufficiency and minimizing the gonadotoxic effect of treatments, temporary ovarian suppression with GnRHa during chemotherapy should not be considered an equivalent or alternative option for fertility preservation, but it should be proposed after embryo and oocyte cryopreservation. Temporary ovarian suppression during chemotherapy achieved by administering a GnRHa is the only strategy that has entered clinical use [55].

9.5 Life After Treatment

Although current oncofertility guidelines are universal among different tumor types and patient profiles, potential disparities between patients due to age, chemotherapy agents employed, and the malignancy itself may also interfere with fertility preservation practices. Consequently, a more methodical investigation of fertility preservation strategies, considering the above parameters, is required, in order to adequately establish the most efficient practices for each patient group.

At the time of diagnosis, a significant proportion of post-pubertal patients have not completed their family planning and express a desire for pregnancy after treatment. Fertility depends on the female's stage in life (before or after puberty, before or after menopause), menstrual history, hormone levels, the type of cancer and treatment, and the treatment doses. Post-treatment pregnancy rates are highly dependent on the type of cancer, with the lowest rates reported for men with a history of acute leukemia or non-Hodgkin's lymphoma and for women with a history of breast or cervical cancer.

Because all these factors need to be considered, it can be hard to predict if a woman is likely to be fertile after chemotherapy. The feasibility and safety of using assisted reproductive technology (ART) following anticancer treatment are an important issue to be considered for adult cancer survivors who did not have access to fertility preservation strategies at the time of diagnosis and/or where there are difficulties with spontaneous conception. Female adult cancer survivors have a higher likelihood of undergoing fertility treatments compared with healthy women, with increasing use over time.

Funding No external funding has been received for the preparation of this chapter.

Disclosure No disclosure to declare.

References

1. Bray F, Ferlay J, Soerjomataram I, Siegel RL, Torre LA, Jemal A. Global cancer statistics 2018: GLOBOCAN estimates of incidence and mortality worldwide for 36 cancers in 185 countries. CA Cancer J Clin. 2018;68(6):394–424. https://doi.org/10.3322/caac.21492. Epub 2018 Sep 12
2. Szabo RA, Marino JL, Hickey M. Managing menopausal symptoms after cancer. Climacteric. 2019;22:572. https://doi.org/10.1080/13697137.2019.1646718.
3. Lambertini M, Peccatori FA, Demeestere I, Amant F, Wyns C, Stukenborg JB, Paluch-Shimon S, Halaska MJ, Uzan C, Meissner J, von Wolff M, Anderson RA, Jordan K, ESMO guidelines Committee. Electronic address: clinicalguidelines@esmo.org. Fertility preservation and post-treatment pregnancies in post-pubertal cancer patients: ESMO Clinical Practice Guidelines†. Ann Oncol. 2020;31(12):1664–78. https://doi.org/10.1016/j.annonc.2020.09.006. Epub 2020 Sep 22

4. Howard-Anderson J, Ganz PA, Bower JE, Stanton AL. Quality of life, fertility concerns, and behavioral health outcomes in younger breast cancer survivors: a systematic review. J Natl Cancer Inst. 2012;104(5):386–405. https://doi.org/10.1093/jnci/djr541. Epub 2012 Jan 23

5. Ruddy KJ, Gelber SI, Tamimi RM, Ginsburg ES, Schapira L, Come SE, Borges VF, Meyer ME, Partridge AH. Prospective study of fertility concerns and preservation strategies in young women with breast cancer. J Clin Oncol. 2014;32(11):1151–6. https://doi.org/10.1200/JCO.2013.52.8877. Epub 2014 Feb 24

6. Partridge AH, Gelber S, Peppercorn J, Sampson E, Knudsen K, Laufer M, Rosenberg R, Przypyszny M, Rein A, Winer EP. Web-based survey of fertility issues in young women with breast cancer. J Clin Oncol. 2004;22(20):4174–83. https://doi.org/10.1200/JCO.2004.01.159. PMID: 15483028

7. Llarena NC, Estevez SL, Tucker SL, Jeruss JS. Impact of fertility concerns on tamoxifen initiation and persistence. J Natl Cancer Inst. 2015;107(10):djv202. https://doi.org/10.1093/jnci/djv202. PMID: 26307641; PMCID: PMC5825683

8. King JW, Davies MC, Roche N, Abraham JM, Jones AL. Fertility preservation in women undergoing treatment for breast cancer in the UK: a questionnaire study. Oncologist. 2012;17:910–6.

9. Zavos A, Valachis A. Risk of chemotherapy-induced amenorrhea in patients with breast cancer: a systematic review and meta-analysis. Acta Oncol. 2016;55(6):664–70. https://doi.org/10.3109/0284186X.2016.1155738. Epub 2016 Apr 22. PMID: 27105082

10. Bines J, Oleske DM, Cobleigh MA. Ovarian function in premenopausal women treated with adjuvant chemotherapy for breast cancer. J Clin Oncol. 1996;14(5):1718–29. https://doi.org/10.1200/JCO.1996.14.5.1718. PMID: 8622093

11. Sukumvanich P, Case LD, Van Zee K, Singletary SE, Paskett ED, Petrek JA, Naftalis E, Naughton MJ. Incidence and time course of bleeding after long-term amenorrhea after breast cancer treatment: a prospective study. Cancer. 2010;116(13):3102–11. https://doi.org/10.1002/cncr.25106. PMID: 20564648

12. Han HS, Ro J, Lee KS, Nam BH, Seo JA, Lee DH, Lee H, Lee ES, Kang HS, Kim SW. Analysis of chemotherapy-induced amenorrhea rates by three different anthracycline and taxane containing regimens for early breast cancer. Breast Cancer Res Treat. 2009;115(2):335–42. https://doi.org/10.1007/s10549-008-0071-9. Epub 2008 May 28. PMID: 18506620

13. Decanter C, Morschhauser F, Pigny P, Lefebvre C, Gallo C, Dewailly D. Anti-Mullerian hormone follow-up in young women treated by chemotherapy for lymphoma: preliminary results. Reprod Biomed Online. 2010;20:280–5.

14. Peigné M, Decanter C. Serum AMH level as a marker of acute and long-term effects of chemotherapy on the ovarian follicular content: a systematic review. Reprod Biol Endocrinol. 2014;12:26. https://doi.org/10.1186/1477-7827-12-26. PMID: 24666685; PMCID: PMC3987687

15. Spears N, Lopes F, Stefansdottir A, Rossi V, De Felici M, Anderson RA, Klinger FG. Ovarian damage from chemotherapy and current approaches to its protection. Hum Reprod Update. 2019;25(6):673–93. https://doi.org/10.1093/humupd/dmz027. PMID: 31600388; PMCID: PMC6847836

16. Lambertini M, Campbell C, Bines J, Korde LA, Izquierdo M, Fumagalli D, Del Mastro L, Ignatiadis M, Pritchard K, Wolff AC, Jackisch C, Lang I, Untch M, Smith I, Boyle F, Xu B, Barrios CH, Baselga J, Moreno-Aspitia A, Piccart M, Gelber RD, de Azambuja E. Adjuvant anti-HER2 therapy, treatment-related amenorrhea, and survival in premenopausal HER2-positive early breast cancer patients. J Natl Cancer Inst. 2019;111(1):86–94. https://doi.org/10.1093/jnci/djy094.

17. Zhao J, Liu J, Chen K, Li S, Wang Y, Yang Y, Deng H, Jia W, Rao N, Liu Q, Su F. What lies behind chemotherapy-induced amenorrhea for breast cancer patients: a meta-analysis. Breast Cancer Res Treat. 2014;145(1):113–28. https://doi.org/10.1007/s10549-014-2914-x. Epub 2014 Mar 27. PMID: 24671358

18. Dezellus A, Barriere P, Campone M, Lemanski C, Vanlemmens L, Mignot L, Delozier T, Levy C, Bendavid C, Debled M, Bachelot T, Jouannaud C, Loustalot C, Mouret-Reynier MA, Gallais-Umbert A, Masson D, Freour T. Prospective evaluation of serum anti-Müllerian hormone dynamics in 250 women of reproductive age treated with chemotherapy for breast cancer. Eur J Cancer. 2017;79:72–80. https://doi.org/10.1016/j.ejca.2017.03.035. Epub 2017 Apr 29. PMID: 28463758

19. Morgan S, Anderson RA, Gourley C, Wallace WH, Spears N. How do chemotherapeutic agents damage the ovary? Hum Reprod Update. 2012;18(5):525–35. https://doi.org/10.1093/humupd/dms022. Epub 2012 May 30

20. Letourneau JM, Ebbel EE, Katz PP, Katz A, Ai WZ, Chien AJ, Melisko ME, Cedars MI, Rosen MP. Pretreatment fertility counseling and fertility preservation improve quality of life in reproductive age women with cancer. Cancer. 2012;118(6):1710–7. https://doi.org/10.1002/cncr.26459. Epub 2011 Sep 1

21. De Vos M, Smitz J, Woodruff TK. Fertility preservation in women with cancer. Lancet. 2014;384(9950):1302–10. https://doi.org/10.1016/S0140-6736(14)60834-5. Erratum in: Lancet 2015 Mar 7;385(9971):856. PMID: 25283571; PMCID: PMC4270060

22. Wallace WH, Thomson AB, Saran F, Kelsey TW. Predicting age of ovarian failure after radiation to a field that includes the ovaries. Int J Radiat Oncol Biol Phys. 2005;62(3):738–44. https://doi.org/10.1016/j.ijrobp.2004.11.038. PMID: 15936554

23. Decanter C, Morschhauser F, Pigny P, Lefebvre C, Gallo C, Dewailly D. Anti-Müllerian hormone follow-up in young women treated by chemotherapy for lymphoma: preliminary results. Reprod Biomed Online. 2010;20(2):280–5. https://doi.org/10.1016/j.rbmo.2009.11.010. Epub 2009 Dec 3

24. Brougham MF, Crofton PM, Johnson EJ, Evans N, Anderson RA, Wallace WH. Anti-Müllerian hormone is a marker of gonadotoxicity in pre- and postpubertal girls treated for cancer: a prospective study. J Clin Endocrinol Metab. 2012;97(6):2059–67. https://doi.org/10.1210/jc.2011-3180. Epub 2012 Apr 3. PMID: 22472563

25. Kalich-Philosoph L, Roness H, Carmely A, Fishel-Bartal M, Ligumsky H, Paglin S, Wolf I, Kanety H, Sredni B, Meirow D. Cyclophosphamide triggers follicle activation and "burnout"; AS101 prevents follicle loss and preserves fertility. Sci Transl Med. 2013;5(185):185ra62. https://doi.org/10.1126/scitranslmed.3005402. PMID: 23677591

26. Cui W, Stern C, Hickey M, Goldblatt F, Anazodo A, Stevenson WS, Phillips KA. Preventing ovarian failure associated with chemotherapy. Med J Aust. 2018;209(9):412–6. https://doi.org/10.5694/mja18.00190. PMID: 30376664

27. Mauri D, Gazouli I, Zarkavelis G, Papadaki A, Mavroeidis L, Gkoura S, Ntellas P, Amylidi AL, Tsali L, Kampletsas E. Chemotherapy associated ovarian failure. Front Endocrinol (Lausanne). 2020;11:572388. https://doi.org/10.3389/fendo.2020.572388. PMID: 33363515; PMCID: PMC7753213

28. Roness H, Kashi O, Meirow D. Prevention of chemotherapy-induced ovarian damage. Fertil Steril. 2016;105(1):20–9. https://doi.org/10.1016/j.fertnstert.2015.11.043. Epub 2015 Dec 8. PMID: 26677788

29. Bedoschi G, Navarro PA, Oktay K. Chemotherapy-induced damage to ovary: mechanisms and clinical impact. Future Oncol. 2016;12(20):2333–44. https://doi.org/10.2217/fon-2016-0176. Epub 2016 Jul 12. PMID: 27402553; PMCID: PMC5066134

30. Brännström M, Dahm-Kähler P. Uterus transplantation and fertility preservation. Best Pract Res Clin Obstet Gynaecol. 2019;55:109–16. https://doi.org/10.1016/j.bpobgyn.2018.12.006. Epub 2018 Dec 21. PMID: 30711374

31. Faddy MJ, Gosden RG. A model conforming the decline in follicle numbers to the age of menopause in women. Hum Reprod. 1996;11(7):1484–6. https://doi.org/10.1093/oxfordjournals.humrep.a019422. PMID: 8671489

32. Richardson SJ, Senikas V, Nelson JF. Follicular depletion during the menopausal transition: evidence for accelerated loss and ultimate exhaustion. J Clin Endocrinol Metab. 1987;65(6):1231–7. https://doi.org/10.1210/jcem-65-6-1231. PMID: 3119654

33. Wallace WH, Thomson AB, Kelsey TW. The radiosensitivity of the human oocyte. Hum Reprod. 2003;18(1):117–21. https://doi.org/10.1093/humrep/deg016. PMID: 12525451

34. Wallace WH, Anderson R, Baird D. Preservation of fertility in young women treated for cancer. Lancet Oncol. 2004;5(5):269–70. https://doi.org/10.1016/S1470-2045(04)01462-7. PMID: 15120661

35. Chang K, Merideth MA, Stratton P. Hormone use for therapeutic amenorrhea and contraception during hematopoietic cell transplantation. Obstet Gynecol. 2015;126(4):779–84. https://doi.org/10.1097/AOG.0000000000001031. PMID: 26348182; PMCID: PMC4580508

36. Kirkham YA, Ornstein MP, Aggarwal A. McQuillan S. No. 313-menstrual suppression in special circumstances. J Obstet Gynaecol Can. 2019;41(2):e7–e17. https://doi.org/10.1016/j.jogc.2018.11.030. PMID: 30638562

37. American College of Obstetricians and Gynecologists' Committee on Adolescent Health Care. Options for prevention and management of menstrual bleeding in adolescent patients undergoing cancer treatment: ACOG Committee Opinion, Number 817. Obstet Gynecol. 2021;137(1):e7–e15. https://doi.org/10.1097/AOG.0000000000004209. PMID: 33399429

38. Poorvu PD, Barton SE, Duncan CN, London WB, Laufer MR, Lehmann LE, Marcus KJ. Use and effectiveness of gonadotropin-releasing hormone agonists for prophylactic menstrual suppression in postmenarchal women who undergo hematopoietic cell transplantation. J Pediatr Adolesc Gynecol. 2016;29(3):265–8. https://doi.org/10.1016/j.jpag.2015.10.013. Epub 2015 Oct 23. PMID: 26506031

39. Lhommé C, Brault P, Bourhis JH, Pautier P, Dohollou N, Dietrich PY, Akbar-Zadeh G, Lucas C, Pico JL, Hayat M. Prevention of menstruation with leuprorelin (GnRH agonist) in women undergoing myelosuppressive chemotherapy or radiochemotherapy for hematological malignancies: a pilot study. Leuk Lymphoma. 2001;42(5):1033–41. https://doi.org/10.3109/10428190109097723. PMID: 11697620

40. Screening and management of bleeding disorders in adolescents with heavy menstrual bleeding: ACOG COMMITTEE OPINION, number 785. Obstet Gynecol. 2019;134(3):e71–83. https://doi.org/10.1097/AOG.0000000000003411. PMID: 31441825

41. ACOG committee opinion no. 557: management of acute abnormal uterine bleeding in nonpregnant reproductive-aged women. Obstet Gynecol. 2013;121(4):891–6. https://doi.org/10.1097/01.AOG.0000428646.67925.9a. PMID: 23635706

42. Tsampras N, Gould D, Fitzgerald CT. Double ovarian stimulation (DuoStim) protocol for fertility preservation in female oncology patients. Hum Fertil. 2017;20(4):248–53.

43. Oktay K, Turan V, Bedoschi G, et al. Fertility preservation success subsequent to concurrent aromatase inhibitor treatment and ovarian stimulation in women with breast cancer. J Clin Oncol. 2015;33(22):2424–9.

44. Practice Committee of the American Society for Reproductive Medicine. Electronic address: asrm@asrm.org. Fertility preservation in patients undergoing gonadotoxic therapy or gonadectomy: a committee opinion. Fertil Steril. 2019;112(6):1022–33. https://doi.org/10.1016/j.fertnstert.2019.09.013. PMID: 31843073

45. Diaz-Garcia C, Domingo J, Garcia-Velasco JA, Herraiz S, Mirabet V, Iniesta I, Cobo A, Remohí J, Pellicer A. Oocyte vitrification versus ovarian cortex transplantation in fertility preservation for adult women undergoing gonadotoxic treatments: a prospective cohort study. Fertil Steril. 2018;109(3):478–485.e2. https://doi.org/10.1016/j.fertnstert.2017.11.018. Epub 2018 Feb 7. PMID: 29428307

46. Beckmann MW, Dittrich R, Lotz L, van der Ven K, van der Ven HH, Liebenthron J, Korell M, Frambach T, Sütterlin M, Schwab R, Seitz S, Müller A, von Wolff M, Häberlin F, Henes M, Winkler-Crepaz K, Krüssel JS, Germeyer A, Toth B. Fertility protection: complications of surgery and results of removal and transplantation of ovarian tissue. Reprod Biomed Online. 2018;36(2):188–96. https://doi.org/10.1016/j.rbmo.2017.10.109. Epub 2017 Nov 9. PMID: 29198423

47. Irtan S, Orbach D, Helfre S, Sarnacki S. Ovarian transposition in prepubescent and adolescent girls with cancer. Lancet Oncol. 2013;14(13):e601–8. https://doi.org/10.1016/S1470-2045(13)70288-2. PMID: 24275133

48. Gubbala K, Laios A, Gallos I, Pathiraja P, Haldar K, Ind T. Outcomes of ovarian transposition in gynaecological cancers; a systematic review and meta-analysis. J Ovarian Res. 2014;7:69. https://doi.org/10.1186/1757-2215-7-69. PMID: 24995040; PMCID: PMC4080752

49. Caretto M, Simoncini T. The need to reduce gonadotoxicity! Fertility reserve after chemotherapy for gynaecological cancer. Gynecol Endocrinol. 2021;37(6):481–2. https://doi.org/10.1080/09513590.2021.1929153. Epub 2021 May 19

50. Lambertini M, Horicks F, Del Mastro L, Partridge AH, Demeestere I. Ovarian protection with gonadotropin-releasing hormone agonists during chemotherapy in cancer patients: from biological evidence to clinical application. Cancer Treat Rev. 2019;72:65–77. https://doi.org/10.1016/j.ctrv.2018.11.006. Epub 2018 Dec 1. PMID: 30530271

51. Oktay K, Harvey BE, Partridge AH, Quinn GP, Reinecke J, Taylor HS, Wallace WH, Wang ET, Loren AW. Fertility preservation in patients with cancer: ASCO clinical practice guideline update. J Clin Oncol. 2018;36(19):1994–2001. https://doi.org/10.1200/JCO.2018.78.1914. Epub 2018 Apr 5. PMID: 29620997

52. Hyman JH, Tulandi T. Fertility preservation options after gonadotoxic chemotherapy. Clin Med Insights Reprod Health. 2013;7:61–9. https://doi.org/10.4137/CMRH.S10848. PMID: 24453520; PMCID: PMC3888081

53. ESHRE Guideline Group on Female Fertility Preservation, Anderson RA, Amant F, Braat D, D'Angelo A, de Sousa C, Lopes SM, Demeestere I, Dwek S, Frith L, Lambertini M, Maslin C, Moura-Ramos M, Nogueira D, Rodriguez-Wallberg K, Vermeulen N. ESHRE guideline: female fertility preservation. Hum Reprod Open. 2020;2020(4):hoaa052. https://doi.org/10.1093/hropen/hoaa052. PMID: 33225079; PMCID: PMC7666361

54. Lee JH, Choi YS. The role of gonadotropin-releasing hormone agonists in female fertility preservation. Clin Exp Reprod Med. 2021;48(1):11–26. https://doi.org/10.5653/cerm.2020.04049. Epub 2021 Feb 18. PMID: 33648041; PMCID: PMC7943347

55. Floyd JL, Campbell S, Rauh-Hain JA, Woodard T. Fertility preservation in women with early-stage gynecologic cancer: optimizing oncologic and reproductive outcomes. Int J Gynecol Cancer. 2021;31(3):345–51. https://doi.org/10.1136/ijgc-2020-001328. Epub 2020 Jun 21. PMID: 32565487

Menorrhagia and the Menopausal Transition

**Amparo Carrasco-Catena, Orly Morgan,
Rocío Belda-Montesinos, and Antonio Cano**

1 Introduction

Menopause is a phenomenon that consists of the definitive cessation of menstruation due to the exhaustion of the follicles in the ovary. At a certain age, all women will undergo menopause. The World Health Organization defines natural menopause as confirmed when amenorrhea is established for at least 1 year in the absence of other physiological or pathological causes [1]. Primary ovarian insufficiency (POI), also known as premature menopause or premature ovarian failure, occurs when menopause takes place before the age of 40. This occurs in approximately 1% of the population.

The process of follicular proliferation takes place only during fetal life and results in a finite amount of follicles in the ovary. The progressive consumption of follicles begins with the intermittent activation of cohorts, which grow and, in most cases, end up degenerating in a process known as follicular atresia. One among the follicles of each cohort will continue to ovulation, upon which they have reached their full development.

A. Carrasco-Catena
Clinical Area Women's Health, Hospital Universitario y Politécnico La Fe, Valencia, Spain

O. Morgan
Department of Medicine and Department of Public Health Sciences,
University of Miami Miller School of Medicine, Miami, FL, USA
e-mail: oxm229@med.miami.edu

R. Belda-Montesinos · A. Cano (✉)
Service of Obstetrics and Gynecology, Hospital General Universitario, Valencia, Spain

Department of Pediatrics, Obstetrics and Gynecology, University of Valencia, Valencia, Spain
e-mail: antonio.cano@uv.es

A. R. Genazzani et al. (eds.), *Menstrual Bleeding and Pain Disorders from Adolescence to Menopause*, ISGE Series,
https://doi.org/10.1007/978-3-031-55300-4_13

The literature is still uncertain as to why some follicles will make it to maturity with ovulation as opposed to others. However the hypothesis exists that it may be linked to differential sensitivity among follicles which results in their different responses to maturity and ovulatory stimulating agents. A progressive inverse selection of the less sensitive follicles is therefore a consequence, which deepens over time. This phenomenon possibly influences the reduction of fertility in the last years of ovarian life, as well as the endocrine deficiencies that follow soon after. These biological mechanisms are the base of menopausal clinical characteristics, such as irregularities in menstrual pattern or other symptoms. That being said, the size of these changes differs between women, which determines that the clinical trajectories that lead to menopause are diverse.

2 The Staging of Reproductive Aging Workshop (STRAW)

The process of follicle exhaustion manifests initially as subclinical changes. As the process continues, the ovaries will reduce hormonal production, and this will further exacerbate problems of follicle growth and maturation with each cycle. These late stages may generate clinical symptoms, i.e., menstrual disturbances in women.

The need to standardize follicular and ovarian hormonal changes of aging moved a group of experts from different scientific societies to promote the Staging of Reproductive Aging Workshop (STRAW) initiative in 2001 [2]. The purpose of STRAW was to obtain a consensus on the different stages detectable along the reproductive lifespan of women. The STRAW initiative evaluated both menstrual features and their corresponding hormonal biological mechanisms. Menopausal symptoms were also included when present. The document was revised and updated in 2012, and the STRAW+10 document was issued [3].

The evidence supporting staging the biological events in a woman's later reproductive years came from consistent data arising from important epidemiological studies: the Study of Women Across the Nation (SWAN) [4], the TREMIN Research Program on Women's Health which is now the oldest ongoing study of menstruation in the world [5], the Melbourne Women's Midlife Health Project [6], as well as the Seattle Midlife Women's Health Project [7].

The reproductive span of women was divided into three broad phases, reproductive, menopausal transition, and postmenopause. Then each of the three was divided into stages, bringing the total to ten and focusing on the final menstrual period.

Importantly, STRAW defined menopausal transition as the term referring to depreciation of ovarian function prior to the diagnosis of menopause and its accompanying hormonal and clinical state.

Each step in STRAW is supported by three types of criteria, defined as principal, supportive, and descriptive, respectively. The principal criteria is the menstrual pattern in all stages, while the supportive criteria includes hormone levels and follicular features. The follicular features would be quantified as the number of antral follicles identified by ultrasound antral follicle count (AFC). They also added descriptive characteristics of the associated clinical symptoms when they are present.

2.1 The Reproductive Phase

The three stages, *early*, *peak*, and *late*, can each have variable duration and as a combined sum make up the reproductive phase (Fig. 1). The transition from early to peak to late results from the mechanisms of follicle exhaustion described above. Individual differences in the timing of stages can be attributed to a number of factors, including the initial pool of follicles, variation in the efficacy of follicle recruitment with each follicular phase, or other potential mechanisms.

The *early stage* initiates with menarche and is only defined by the menstrual pattern, which is either regular or irregular. The variability at this stage is due to the high prevalence of menstrual irregularity in the initial cycles following menarche [8].

The *peak stage* has regular menstrual cycles with normal values of follicle-stimulating hormone (FSH). This hormone is the gonadotropin responsible for promoting the growth of the follicles in the cohort, already from the end of the previous cycle, when the corpus luteum is suffering a progressively reduced hormonal activity. Anti-Mullerian hormone (AMH) is an important hormone marker during this period as it correlates with ovarian reserve and fertility [9] and trends downward with age.

The *late stage* includes two different steps, which slightly differ in menstrual pattern as well as in their underlying physiological hormone patterns.

In the first step, the individual still maintains regular menstrual cycles; however there is a decrease in AMH levels. Decreased AMH indicates the progressively diminished ovarian reserve at this period and the subsequent fall in fertility even with regular menstrual cycles. This information is insightful because AMH is produced by the growing follicles, and not by those at rest [10]. Decreasing AMH levels correlate with the progressive reduction in the number of growing follicles in each cohort and can be viewed as a predictor for the number of follicles still residing in the ovary. The AFC detected by ultrasound is also low, in consistence with the AMH levels.

The second step may include small changes in menstrual periods, which may become shorter and/or have a change in flow pattern. Hormonally the individual may exhibit small changes in FSH which will now have slight increases in the initiation of the follicular phase. Inhibin B is another hormone that can be trended, as it will decrease as the stage progresses.

Inhibin B is a protein heterodimer, composed of two monomeric sub-units, α and β_B, linked by a single disulfide bond. The reduction in the ovarian output of inhibin B, a specific inhibitor of the synthesis and release of FSH, is a key mechanism determining the observed increase of FSH [11]. Higher FSH levels then stimulate

MENARCHE

FMP (0)

Stage	−5	−4	−3b	−3a	−2	−1	+1a	+1b	+1c	+2
Terminology	REPRODUCTIVE				MENOPAUSAL TRANSITION		POSTMENOPAUSE			
	Early	Peak	Late		Early	Late	Early			Late
					Perimenopause					
Duration	Variable				Variable	1–3 years	2 years (1+1)		3–6 years	Remaining lifespan
PRINCIPAL CRITERIA										
Menstrual Cycle	Variable to regular	Regular	Regular	Subtle changes in Flow/Length	Variable Length Persistent ≥7-day difference in length of consecutive cycles	Interval of amenorrhea of ≥60 days				
SUPPORTIVE CRITERIA										
Endocrine FSH			Low	Variable[a]	↑ Variable[a]	↑ >25 IU/L[b]	↑ Variable[a]		Stabilizes	
AMH			Low	Low	Low	Low	Low		Very low	
Inhibin B				Low	Low	Low	Low		Very low	
Antral Follicle Count			Low	Low	Low	Low	Very low		Very low	
DESCRIPTIVE CHARACTERISTICS										
Symptoms						Vasomotor symptoms Likely	Vasomotor symptoms Most Likely			Increasing symptoms of urogenital artophy

Fig. 1 The Stages of the Reproductive Aging Workshop +10 (STRAW +10). [a]Blood draw on cycle days 2–5. ↑ = elevated. [b]Approximate expected level based on assays using current international pituitary standard. Figure is a modification of work found in Harlow et al. [[3]]. (With permission from [3]. Copyright conveyed through Rights Link)

increased levels of follicle growth completing follicular development earlier in the cycle, usually 1–5 days sooner [12].

FSH stimulates estradiol (E2) production in granulosa cells, but whether the process is accompanied by an increase in the output of E2 is a matter of debate in the literature [11, 13]. The increase in E2 levels found by some investigators [11] fits poorly with the reduction in granulosa cells that occurs with age. However the over-stimulation provided by the increase in FSH, particularly in the setting of increased aromatase activity [13], appears to support E2 production despite the depreciation in granulosa cells.

2.2 *The Menopausal Transition Phase*

STRAW divides the menopausal transition phase into two stages, early and late, coded as -2 and -1 (Fig. 1). Both are variable in length, but while the early stage was not given a limit, the late stage was categorized as lasting for 1–3 years. The menopausal transition almost overlaps the traditional term of "perimenopause." The difference is that perimenopause includes the first year after menopause.

The hallmark of the menopausal transition is that it is often symptomatic. Many women will complain of cycle irregularity during this transition, in which periods of amenorrhea may alternate with heavy bleeding episodes, as well as symptoms like hot flashes, mood changes, premenstrual cramping, etc.

Epidemiological studies have found that this characteristic pattern of menstrual disturbances progressively evolves to permanent amenorrhea. The incidence of anovulatory cycles increases in parallel with that trend in the menstrual pattern. A prospective study conducted over 4 years involving 250 Australian women ages 45–55 yielded important insight into the variability of the menopausal transition period. The study found that 30% of the women reported no change when comparing the last 3 months with the previous 12 months, 10% of the women reported change in bleeding frequency but not amount, 22% reported change in amount but not frequency, 26% reported change in both frequency and amount, and 12% reported 3 or more months of amenorrhea [14]. Moreover, a sub-cohort of the SWAN study was followed until their last menstrual period (LMP) or up to 10 years, whichever came first. Basic hormones were investigated together with the menstrual pattern once per year. Anovulatory cycles increased as the LMP was approaching [15]. Two types of anovulatory cycles were described, those linked with bleeding, in which there was an association with the levels of estrogens, and those linked with amenorrhea, in which the menopausal pattern of low estrogens and high FSH and luteinizing hormone (LH) was increasingly prevalent [16].

2.2.1 The Early Stage

A ≥7-day difference in length of consecutive menstrual cycles defines the early stage of the menopausal transition. This stage has a variable duration.

Endocrinologically, the pattern of the previous -3a stage (Fig. 1) was more pronounced, so that the elevation of FSH at the initiation of the cycle is more intensely prevalent, as is the level of reduction in AMH and inhibin B. Sometimes they may be even below detection limits. AFC continues to be low.

A reduced activity of the corpus luteum, with a slightly diminished excretion of progesterone and inhibin A, has been suggested as a factor contributing to the increase in FSH [16]. The mechanism for this is unclear, although reduction of follicular quality has been suggested [17]. The rise in FSH has already occurred by the luteal phase, and follicle recruitment takes place prior to onset of menses. During one cycle, the hormones may compound to cause the growth of the next cycle's dominant follicle to occur during the luteal phase, and its ovulation may happen soon after menses [18].

The high FSH level may induce intervals of high estrogenic output, which may alternate with other periods of hypoestrogenism. Clinically, the upward trend of anovulatory cycles continues and may become as high as 10–15% [15]. The fairly high prevalence of appreciable levels of estrogens makes the abnormal bleeding episodes anticipated. Menopausal symptoms, like hot flashes or irritability, appear as a consequence of hypoestrogenic intervals, although they are more frequent in the next -1 stage. The feeling of bloating can also occur in the setting of the hyperestrogenic interludes.

2.2.2 The Late Stage

Women enter this stage, coded as -1, when amenorrhea has lasted for at least 60 days. The average duration of this stage is 1–3 years.

Endocrinologically, this phase consists of a definitive reduction in the number of follicles and the decrease in their quality. This further contributes to the increase in FSH and lower estrogen levels, although some fluctuation can still be found for unclear reasons. The rate of amenorrheic anovulation progressively increases as the stage goes on (Table 1).

Table 1 Features of the late stage of the menopausal transition according to SWAN [15, 16]

Ovulatory cycles	Decline (from 80.9% to 64.7%)	
Anovulatory (bleeding)		
	Estrogens	= or slightly ↓
	FSH	↑
Anovulatory nonbleeding		
	Estrogens	↓↓
	FSH	↑↑

FSH follicle-stimulating hormone

Menopausal symptoms, e.g., hot flashes, irritability, poor sleep, etc., will appear more frequently as a result of the increasing hypoestrogenic periods, and symptoms associated with hyper-estrogenism will slowly fade.

Anovulation may also be influenced by the central nervous system, the hypothalamus and pituitary, which are involved in both the negative and positive feedback of estrogens in the normal cycle. This phenomenon has been deeply investigated in rodents [19] and has been confirmed to also be the case for humans [20, 21]. The size of the impact regarding this phenomenon in clinical settings is still elusive.

3 Clinical Approach

3.1 Diagnosis

As for any uterine bleeding disorder, the PALM-COEIN acronym proposed by FIGO (International Federation of Gynecology and Obstetrics) continues to be in use. PALM stands for polyp, adenomyosis, leiomyoma, and malignancy, while COEIN stands for coagulopathy, ovulatory dysfunction, endometrial, iatrogenic, and not yet classified [22]. Women in menopausal transition are at the end of their reproductive period, and pathologies related to reproductive activity, such as leiomyomatosis, adenomyosis, or malignancy, are more prevalent. Anovulatory cycles, and specifically those with good estrogen levels, should be considered in the differential diagnosis of abnormal bleeding.

A review on the topic indicates that a detailed systematic diagnostic approach needs to be followed in order to cover the array of potential situations of clinical interest [23].

Taking a detailed medical history is a must. It may provide some hints which may be particularly helpful in determining differential diagnoses. For example, abnormal bleeding consisting of heavy flow, but regular in the timing of the cycle, is consistent with pathologies like leiomyoma or adenomyosis, but rarely due to malignancy.

Along with the history and physical exam, including pelvic and speculum examination, four main objectives should be taken into account: (i) elucidation of the ovulatory status of the cycle, (ii) laboratory values, (iii) imaging techniques, and (iv) endometrial histology.

A basic laboratory evaluation should include the assessment of hemostatic disorders, although in most cases they manifest early in life and are diagnosed in association with profuse bleeding in adolescence [24]. The resulting anemia or iron insufficiency should be shown by hematological and iron studies, particularly when bleeding disturbances are present for weeks or months. Also, two frequent clinical situations need to be ruled out, pregnancy for which a HCG test will be required and thyroid pathology.

Imaging techniques are crucial to find out whether an anatomical abnormality is the root of the problem. Endovaginal ultrasound is the key to detect leiomyomatosis [25], adenomyosis [26], or polyps [27]. The high discriminative potential of modern ultrasound probes has taken the term "sonomicroscopy," since they measure endometrial thickness with millimetric accuracy, and, as such, a normal thin endometrium in postmenopausal bleeding has higher negative predictive value for endometrial cancer than blind endometrial sampling [23].

Work-up for the differential diagnosis of polyps and thickened endometrium may require the use of saline infusion sonography (SIS), an easy-to-use technique that involves projecting fluid into the uterine cavity to obtain a detailed view of existing structures, including a polyp, if present [28].

A histological diagnosis is necessary when the cause of abnormal bleeding is still unclear. Endometrial biopsy can be done via cannular aspiration, and there are several new technologies available on the market which are made to do this. The Cornier cannula is very popular, since it may be used in the office in most cases. However, there is debate about how accurate the system is in providing a reliable diagnosis. The false negative rate was 33% in initial studies where blind aspiration sampling was performed in women with confirmed endometrial carcinoma [29]. The inaccuracies were more frequent when the process was localized to less than 50% of the surface. Although the data was only proven in studies with a small sample size, a Practice Bulletin of the American College of Obstetricians and Gynecologists stated that blind aspiration biopsy was reliable in the diagnosis of endometrial cancer only when an adequate specimen was obtained and when the process was global [30].

Hysteroscopy has been proposed as an alternative to disclose whether there is a structural abnormality, such as polyps or intracavitary leiomyomas. While this information may be also provided by SIS, the potential to selectively biopsy an abnormal area may be an advantage. The design of new sets allowing for the practice of the technique in the office, without the requirement of anesthesia, has contributed to the popularity of the technique, although the cost is still a barrier to use. One strength of hysteroscopy is the high specificity (92–95%) and reasonable sensitivity (78–98%) for endometrial pathological diagnosis, but in some postmenopausal women, the procedure may be technically difficult to perform [31]. The possibility of spreading malignant cells into the abdomen due to the positive inflation pressure has been a matter of concern, although small studies suggest it does not seem to influence the prognosis [31].

3.2   Management

Clinicians should keep in mind that while anovulation due to persistent estrogenic stimulation is expected in most cases, bleeding may be due to other causes. This has been addressed above, and specific management needs to be considered in case of pregnancy, malignancy, or structural pathology, such as polyps, leiomyoma, etc.

Anovulation linked with persistent estrogen stimulation causes increased proliferation resulting in hyperplastic endometrium, a high prevalence condition. An observational study on 119 endometrial samples from women older than 40 with abnormal uterine bleeding reported that the histopathological diagnosis was proliferative endometrium in 34% and endometrial hyperplasia in 24%. No endometrial carcinoma was found [32].

The goals of treatment should include (i) reduction of blood loss when heavy or having a clinical impact, (ii) regulation of the menstrual cycle, (iii) reassurance of the patient by making it clear that this is a frequent event during the menopausal transition, and (iv) improving quality of life [23].

Expectant treatment may be a possibility when the impact of bleeding is small and the patient is confident and satisfied with the option.

Otherwise, there is a wide range of management options available for abnormal bleeding, and the work-up and treatment should be tailored to the individual wants and needs of the patient. Since the menopausal transition state involves high rates of estrogen-induced proliferative and hyperplastic endometrium, progestogen is a preferential option for hormonal treatment. Other medical alternatives should also be considered before entering the surgical pathway.

3.2.1 Progestogens

The wide array of progestogens needs to be critically evaluated for their metabolic and oncologic impact. A good option is the use of micronized progesterone or dydrogesterone, because both have preferential affinity by the progesterone receptor, with little interaction with other steroidal receptors, like androgen receptor, glucocorticoid receptors, or mineralocorticoid receptors [33]. Moreover, their impact on the risk of breast cancer is considered low [34]. The efficacy in terms of endometrial protection or bleeding control is considered acceptable for both compounds [35–38]. Moreover, micronized progesterone may be given as a localized vaginal suppository and therefore is an alternative which will have low circulating levels and little systemic effect [37].

Other progestogens have been considered more powerful in experimental analyses [39]. Medroxyprogesterone acetate has been used for many years with good results in women bleeding during the menopausal transition [40].

The intrauterine device containing levo-norgestrel (LNG-IUD) deserves a specific comment. Originally designed for contraceptive use, its effectiveness has been subsequently shown for the control of heavy menstrual bleeding, endometrial hyperplasia, and as the progestogenic component in menopausal hormone therapy [41]. Indeed, its effectiveness at all those targets is at the base of its popularity. A Danish nationwide study between 1996 and 2017 showed a consistent increase in the use by all age ranges and, specifically, that of women in their late reproductive period [42]. Moreover, the ECLIPSE trial confirmed the LNG-IUD as a cost-effective option that increases the quality of life of the user [43]. The systemic impact seems small, although some doubts persist in what regards the increase in the risk of breast cancer [44]. Other long-acting parenteral progestogens, like subcutaneous implants, are also a reasonable option, with a similar effectiveness and risk profile.

Oral hormonal contraceptives, either the progestogenic only pill or the varied options of combined estrogen-progestogen preparations, are a reasonable possibility too. Non-smokers with low cardiovascular risk factors, including venous thrombosis, are preferred when using the combined preparations.

3.2.2 Surgery

This is generally considered an alternative second-line therapy after trials of medical treatment, although some women may feel inclined to take it as a primary option. In the menopausal transition, fertility is not usually a variable in analysis of patient priorities, which makes surgical management an attractive solution because it is viewed as a definitive cure. However, while this is the case of hysterectomy, it is not necessarily that of the other procedures, for example, endometrial ablation. That being said, the advances in techniques mean that these procedures can be performed quickly and with light anesthesia, in an outpatient surgical center, and therefore there is increased interest in them.

A systematic review of eight RCT has compared effectiveness, acceptability, and safety of techniques of endometrial ablation by any means versus hysterectomy by any means for the treatment of heavy menstrual bleeding [45]. Authors concluded that both alternatives achieved a high rate of satisfaction, but hysterectomy involved longer operating time and recovery as well as a higher rate of postoperative complications. Endometrial ablation, on the other hand, failed more frequently after initial treatment, which involved higher rates of repeat surgery [46].

4 Conclusion

The menopausal transition is a crucial stage in the late reproductive period of women. The steps followed during this phase are stratified in the STRAW initiative. Some women may have significant clinical symptoms affecting health and quality of life at certain stages. Bleeding disturbances are one principal feature, which needs attention for both diagnosis and management. Some severe pathologies, mainly malignancy, need to be ruled out, and, even if not present, the amount and/or persistence of the bleeding deserves attention.

References

1. World Health Organization. WHO Scientific Group on Research on the Menopause in the 1990s. WHO Technical Report Series. Genevad: WHO; 1996. http://apps.who.int/iris/bitstream/10665/41841/1/WHO_TRS_866.pdf. Accessed 27Aug 2022
2. Soules MR, Sherman S, Parrott E, Rebar R, Santoro N, Utian W, et al. Executive summary: Stages of Reproductive Aging Workshop (STRAW). Fertil Steril. 2001;76:874–8.
3. Harlow S, Gass M, Hall JE, Lobo R, Maki P, Rebar RW, et al. Executive summary of the Stages of Reproductive Aging Workshop + 10: addressing the unfinished agenda of staging reproductive aging. Fertil Steril. 2012;97:843–51.
4. Gold EB, Sternfeld B, Kelsey JL, Brown C, Mouton C, Reame N, Salamone L, Stellato R. Relation of demographic and lifestyle factors to symptoms in a multi-racial/ethnic population of women 40-55 years of age. Am J Epidemiol. 2000;152:463–73. https://doi.org/10.1093/aje/152.5.463. PMID: 10981461
5. Mansfield PK, Carey M, Anderson A, Barsom SH, Koch PB. Staging the menopausal transition: data from the TREMIN Research Program on Women's Health. Womens Health Issues. 2004;14(6):220–6. https://doi.org/10.1016/j.whi.2004.08.002. PMID: 15589772
6. https://researchdata.edu.au/melbourne-womens-midlife-health-project/97876. Accessed 27 Aug 2022.
7. Woods NF, Mitchell ES. The Seattle Midlife Women's Health Study: a longitudinal prospective study of women during the menopausal transition and early postmenopause. Womens Midlife Health. 2016;9(2):6. https://doi.org/10.1186/s40695-016-0019-x. PMID: 30766702; PMCID: PMC6299967
8. Carlson LJ, Shaw ND. Development of ovulatory menstrual cycles in adolescent girls. J Pediatr Adolesc Gynecol. 2019;32(3):249–53. https://doi.org/10.1016/j.jpag.2019.02.119. Epub 2019 Feb 14. PMID: 30772499; PMCID: PMC6570576
9. Moolhuijsen LME, Visser JA. Anti-Müllerian hormone and ovarian reserve: update on assessing ovarian function. J Clin Endocrinol Metab. 2020;105(11):3361–73. https://doi.org/10.1210/clinem/dgaa513. PMID: 32770239; PMCID: PMC7486884
10. Visser JA. Shaping up the function of anti-Müllerian hormone in ovaries of mono-ovulatory species. Hum Reprod. 2016;31(7):1403–5. https://doi.org/10.1093/humrep/dew101. Epub 2016 May 9. PMID: 27165619
11. Welt CK, McNicholl DJ, Taylor AE, Hall JE. Female reproductive aging is marked by decreased secretion of dimeric inhibin. J Clin Endocrinol Metab. 1999;84(1):105–11. https://doi.org/10.1210/jcem.84.1.5381.
12. Klein NA, Battaglia DE, Fujimoto VY, Davis GS, Bremner WJ, Soules MR. Reproductive aging: accelerated ovarian follicular development associated with a monotropic follicle-stimulating hormone rise in normal older women. J Clin Endocrinol Metab. 1996;81(3):1038–45. https://doi.org/10.1210/jcem.81.3.8772573. PMID: 8772573
13. Shaw ND, Srouji SS, Welt CK, Cox KH, Fox JH, Adams JA, Sluss PM, Hall JE. Compensatory increase in ovarian aromatase in older regularly cycling women. J Clin Endocrinol Metab. 2015;100(9):3539–47. https://doi.org/10.1210/JC.2015-2191. Epub 2015 Jun 30. PMID: 26126208; PMCID: PMC4570155
14. Dudley EC, Hopper JL, Taffe J, Guthrie JR, Burger HG, Dennerstein L. Using longitudinal data to define the perimenopause by menstrual cycle characteristics. Climacteric. 1998;1(1):18–25. https://doi.org/10.3109/13697139809080677.
15. Santoro N, Crawford SL, El Khoudary SR, Allshouse AA, Burnett-Bowie SA, Finkelstein J, Derby C, Matthews K, Kravitz HM, Harlow SD, Greendale GA, Gold EB, Kazlauskaite R, McConnell D, Neal-Perry G, Pavlovic J, Randolph J, Weiss G, Chen HY, Lasley B. Menstrual cycle hormone changes in women traversing menopause: study of women's health across the nation. J Clin Endocrinol Metab. 2017;102(7):2218–29. https://doi.org/10.1210/jc.2016-4017. PMID: 28368525; PMCID: PMC5505186

16. Santoro N, Crawford SL, Lasley WL, Luborsky JL, Matthews KA, McConnell D, Randolph JF Jr, Gold EB, Greendale GA, Korenman SG, Powell L, Sowers MF, Weiss G. Factors related to declining luteal function in women during the menopausal transition. J Clin Endocrinol Metab. 2008;93(5):1711–21. https://doi.org/10.1210/jc.2007-2165. Epub 2008 Feb 19. PMID: 18285413; PMCID: PMC2386686

17. Santoro N, Roeca C, Peters BA, Neal-Perry G. The menopause transition: signs, symptoms, and management options. J Clin Endocrinol Metab. 2021;106(1):1–15. https://doi.org/10.1210/clinem/dgaa764. PMID: 33095879

18. Hale GE, Hughes CL, Burger HG, Robertson DM, Fraser IS. Atypical estradiol secretion and ovulation patterns caused by luteal out-of-phase (LOOP) events underlying irregular ovulatory menstrual cycles in the menopausal transition. Menopause. 2009;16(1):50–9. https://doi.org/10.1097/GME.0b013e31817ee0c2. PMID: 18978637

19. Wise PM. Neuroendocrine ageing: its impact on the reproductive system of the female rat. J Reprod Fertil Suppl. 1993;46:35–46. PMID: 8100275

20. Cano A, Gimeno F, Fuente T, Parrilla JJ, Abad L. The positive feedback of estradiol on gonadotropin secretion in women with perimenopausal dysfunctional uterine bleeding. Eur J Obstet Gynecol Reprod Biol. 1986;22(5–6):353–8. https://doi.org/10.1016/0028-2243(86)90125-5. PMID: 3095159

21. Weiss G, Skurnick JH, Goldsmith LT, Santoro NF, Park SJ. Menopause and hypothalamic-pituitary sensitivity to estrogen. JAMA. 2004;292(24):2991–6. https://doi.org/10.1001/jama.292.24.2991. Erratum in: JAMA. 2005 Jan 12; 293(2): 163. Erratum in: JAMA 2007 Jul 18; 298(3): 288. PMID: 15613667

22. Munro MG, Critchley HO, Broder MS, Fraser IS, FIGO Working Group on Menstrual Disorders. FIGO classification system (PALM-COEIN) for causes of abnormal uterine bleeding in nongravid women of reproductive age. Int J Gynaecol Obstet. 2011;113(1):3–13. https://doi.org/10.1016/j.ijgo.2010.11.011. Epub 2011 Feb 22. PMID: 21345435

23. Goldstein SR, Lumsden MA. Abnormal uterine bleeding in perimenopause. Climacteric. 2017;20(5):414–20. https://doi.org/10.1080/13697137.2017.1358921. Epub 2017 Aug 7. PMID: 28780893

24. Kouides PA, Conard J, Peyvandi F, Lukes A, Kadir R. Hemostasis and menstruation: appropriate investigation for underlying disorders of hemostasis in women with excessive menstrual bleeding. Fertil Steril. 2005;84(5):1345–51. https://doi.org/10.1016/j.fertnstert.2005.05.035. PMID: 16275228

25. Awiwi MO, Badawy M, Shaaban AM, Menias CO, Horowitz JM, Soliman M, Jensen CT, Gaballah AH, Ibarra-Rovira JJ, Feldman MK, Wang MX, Liu PS, Elsayes KM. Review of uterine fibroids: imaging of typical and atypical features, variants, and mimics with emphasis on workup and FIGO classification. Abdom Radiol (NY). 2022;47(7):2468–85. https://doi.org/10.1007/s00261-022-03545-x. Epub 2022 May 13. PMID: 35554629

26. Wong S, Ray CE Jr. Adenomyosis—an overview. Semin Intervent Radiol. 2022;39(1):119–22. https://doi.org/10.1055/s-0042-1742345. PMID: 35210742; PMCID: PMC8856779

27. Vitale SG, Haimovich S, Laganà AS, Alonso L, Di Spiezio SA, Carugno J, From the Global Community of Hysteroscopy Guidelines Committee. Endometrial polyps. An evidence-based diagnosis and management guide. Eur J Obstet Gynecol Reprod Biol. 2021;260:70–7. https://doi.org/10.1016/j.ejogrb.2021.03.017. Epub 2021 Mar 13. PMID: 33756339

28. Kumar S, Nepal P, Narayanasamy S, Khandelwal A, Sapire J, Ojili V. Current update on status of saline infusion sonohysterosalpingography. Abdom Radiol (NY). 2022;47(4):1435–47. https://doi.org/10.1007/s00261-022-03427-2. Epub 2022 Feb 2. PMID: 35112137

29. Ferry J, Farnsworth A, Webster M, Wren B. The efficacy of the pipelle endometrial biopsy in detecting endometrial carcinoma. Aust N Z J Obstet Gynaecol. 1993;33(1):76–8. https://doi.org/10.1111/j.1479-828x.1993.tb02060.x. PMID: 8498946

30. Committee on Practice Bulletins—Gynecology. Practice bulletin no. 128: diagnosis of abnormal uterine bleeding in reproductive-aged women. Obstet Gynecol. 2012;120(1):197–206. https://doi.org/10.1097/AOG.0b013e318262e320. PMID: 22914421

31. Dreisler E, Poulsen LG, Antonsen SL, Ceausu I, Depypere H, Erel CT, Lambrinoudaki I, Pérez-López FR, Simoncini T, Tremollieres F, Rees M, Ulrich LG, European Menopause and Andropause Society. EMAS clinical guide: assessment of the endometrium in peri and postmenopausal women. Maturitas. 2013;75(2):181–90. https://doi.org/10.1016/j.maturitas.2013.03.011. Epub 2013 Apr 22. PMID: 23619009

32. Damle RP, Dravid NV, Suryawanshi KH, Gadre AS, Bagale PS, Ahire N. Clinicopathological spectrum of endometrial changes in peri-menopausal and post-menopausal abnormal uterine bleeding: a 2 years study. J Clin Diagn Res. 2013;7(12):2774–6. https://doi.org/10.7860/JCDR/2013/6291.3755. Epub 2013 Dec 15. PMID: 24551634; PMCID: PMC3919318

33. Stanczyk FZ, Hapgood JP, Winer S, Mishell DR Jr. Progestogens used in postmenopausal hormone therapy: differences in their pharmacological properties, intracellular actions, and clinical effects. Endocr Rev. 2013;34(2):171–208. https://doi.org/10.1210/er.2012-1008. Epub 2012 Dec 13. PMID: 23238854; PMCID: PMC3610676

34. Vinogradova Y, Coupland C, Hippisley-Cox J. Use of hormone replacement therapy and risk of breast cancer: nested case-control studies using the QResearch and CPRD databases. BMJ. 2020;371:m3873. https://doi.org/10.1136/bmj.m3873. PMID: 33115755; PMCID: PMC7592147

35. Affinito P, Di Carlo C, Di Mauro P, Napolitano V, Nappi C. Endometrial hyperplasia: efficacy of a new treatment with a vaginal cream containing natural micronized progesterone. Maturitas. 1994;20(2–3):191–8. https://doi.org/10.1016/0378-5122(94)90016-7. PMID: 7715472

36. Karakus S, Kiran G, Ciralik H. Efficacy of micronised vaginal progesterone versus oral dydrogestrone in the treatment of irregular dysfunctional uterine bleeding: a pilot randomised controlled trial. Aust N Z J Obstet Gynaecol. 2009;49(6):685–8. https://doi.org/10.1111/j.1479-828X.2009.01093.x. PMID: 20070724

37. Fernández-Murga L, Hermenegildo C, Tarín JJ, García-Pérez MÁ, Cano A. Endometrial response to concurrent treatment with vaginal progesterone and transdermal estradiol. Climacteric. 2012;15(5):455–9. https://doi.org/10.3109/13697137.2011.644360. Epub 2012 Feb 9. PMID: 22321028

38. Lobo RA, Archer DF, Kagan R, Kaunitz AM, Constantine GD, Pickar JH, Graham S, Bernick B, Mirkin S. A 17β-estradiol-progesterone Oral capsule for vasomotor symptoms in postmenopausal women: a randomized controlled trial. Obstet Gynecol. 2018;132(1):161–70. https://doi.org/10.1097/AOG.0000000000002645. Erratum in: Obstet Gynecol 2018 Sep; 132(3): 786. PMID: 29889748

39. Sitruk-Ware R. Progestogens in hormonal replacement therapy: new molecules, risks, and benefits. Menopause. 2002;9(1):6–15. https://doi.org/10.1097/00042192-200201000-00003. PMID: 11791081

40. Rezk M, Masood A, Dawood R. Perimenopausal bleeding: patterns, pathology, response to progestins and clinical outcome. J Obstet Gynaecol. 2015;35(5):517–21. https://doi.org/10.3109/01443615.2014.977781. PMID: 25383726

41. Wildemeersch D. Why perimenopausal women should consider to use a levonorgestrel intrauterine system. Gynecol Endocrinol. 2016;32(8):659–61. https://doi.org/10.3109/09513590.2016.1153056. Epub 2016 Mar 1. PMID: 26930021

42. Meaidi A, Kuhr Skals R, Alexander Gerds T, Lidegaard O, Torp-Pedersen C. Decline in Danish use of oral tranexamic acid with increasing use of the levonorgestrel-releasing intrauterine system: a nationwide drug utilization study. Contraception. 2020;101(5):321–6. https://doi.org/10.1016/j.contraception.2019.12.013. Epub 2020 Jan 11. PMID: 31935386

43. Gupta J, Kai J, Middleton L, Pattison H, Gray R, Daniels J, ECLIPSE Trial Collaborative Group. Levonorgestrel intrauterine system versus medical therapy for menorrhagia. N Engl J Med. 2013;368(2):128–37. https://doi.org/10.1056/NEJMoa1204724. PMID: 23301731

44. Mørch LS, Skovlund CW, Hannaford PC, Iversen L, Fielding S, Lidegaard Ø. Contemporary hormonal contraception and the risk of breast cancer. N Engl J Med. 2017;377(23):2228–39. https://doi.org/10.1056/NEJMoa1700732. PMID: 29211679
45. Fergusson RJ, Lethaby A, Shepperd S, Farquhar C. Endometrial resection and ablation versus hysterectomy for heavy menstrual bleeding. Cochrane Database Syst Rev. 2013;11:CD000329. https://doi.org/10.1002/14651858.CD000329.pub2. Update in: Cochrane Database Syst Rev. 2019 Aug 29; 8: CD000329. PMID: 24288154
46. Munro MG. Endometrial ablation. Best Pract Res Clin Obstet Gynaecol. 2018;46:120–39. https://doi.org/10.1016/j.bpobgyn.2017.10.003. Epub 2017 Oct 20. PMID: 29128205

Bleeding Abnormalities During Menopause Hormone Therapy

Frisetti Carpani Vittoria, Andrea Giannini,
Tommaso Simoncini, and Andrea R. Genazzani

1 Introduction

Abnormal uterine bleeding (AUB) is an umbrella term that describes irregular menstrual cycles in frequency, regularity, duration, and flow volume outside pregnancy [1]. One-third of women will experience AUB in their own life, 70% of which occur during peri- and postmenopausal years [2]. Postmenopausal bleeding (PMB) is among the 5% of all gynecological consults [3]. Remarkably, up to 45% of perimenopausal women present PMB due to hormonal imbalance [4]. Nevertheless, a clinical examination, including imaging, laboratory tests, and biopsy, is crucial to exclude other important causes of PMB, such as endometrial polyps, hyperplasia, and carcinoma. Furthermore, there is significant variability in how providers perform diagnostic assessments of AUB. Therefore, this dissertation intends to quantify the prevalence of bleeding abnormalities during menopause hormone therapy (MHT) while also evaluating if any differences in the incidence of PMB related to MHT composition exist. Ultimately, it aspires to take a step forward in exploring the proper diagnostic investigation to exclude endometrial pathologies causing perimenopausal bleeding abnormalities.

F. C. Vittoria · A. Giannini · T. Simoncini · A. R. Genazzani (✉)
Department of Clinical and Experimental Medicine, Division of Obstetrics and Gynecology,
University of Pisa, Pisa, Italy
e-mail: v.frisetticarpani@studenti.unipi.it; andrea.giannini@unipi.it;
tommso.simoncini@unipi.it

A. R. Genazzani et al. (eds.), *Menstrual Bleeding and Pain Disorders from
Adolescence to Menopause*, ISGE Series,
https://doi.org/10.1007/978-3-031-55300-4_14

2 Incidence of Bleeding Abnormalities During Menopause Hormone Therapy

Menopause hormone therapy (MHT) is the most effective therapeutical option approved by the North America Menopause Society (NAMS) and the International Menopause Society (IMS) for women in peri- and postmenopausal age experiencing vasomotor symptoms (VMS), genitourinary syndrome of menopause (GSM), premature ovarian insufficiency (POI), as well as preventing osteoporosis [5]. However, despite the benefits of MHT, women may report side effects, including but not limited to PMBs, with a different frequency rate depending on the woman's period of reproduction, as shown in Table 1. Therefore, bleeding abnormalities can lead to decreased patient compliance and a worsened Quality of Life (QoL) while also requiring diagnostic assessment to exclude PMB as an alarm for other endometrial pathologies. Thus, the goal should be to take preventive action to reduce the percentage of PMBs reported during MHT administration by investigating how the endometrium responds to various hormonal treatment compositions. The first MHT compound included more than ten estrogenic molecules isolated from pregnant mares' urine [6]. In 1 year, a critical study reported a correlation between conjugated estrogens (CEE) and the development of endometrial cancer [7]. Therefore, this increased risk of carcinoma has been overcome by introducing progestogen in patients with an intact uterus. Different combinations of estrogen plus progestogen compounds exist, while numerous sequential- and continuous-combined HT formulations are approved. In the sequential regimen, abnormal bleeding reports a frequency rate of 8–40%. On the other hand, during continuous-combined HT administration, AUB's frequency rate varies from 0% to 77% in the first year [8].

Table 1 Tips and tricks for minimizing bleeding abnormalities during menopause hormone therapy administration

Considering women's reproductive age
Preferring OC/sequential HRT in perimenopause
Preferring CC HRT in postmenopausal
Choose the natural routes of administration
Vaginal (ovarian vessels)
Transdermal
Choose a tailored combination of compounds and the correct dose of molecules
Minimizing estrogen and progestogen doses
Prefer estradiol
Prefer vaginal administration of progesterone

OC oral contraceptive, *CC* continuous combined [5, 12, 13]

The frequency rate of such abnormal bleeding depends on many parameters, including the woman's reproductive age, doses, routes of administration, and duration of MHT. With particular attention to the compounds' composition, estrogen's effect in stimulating endometrial development is already well known as a crucial issue in endometrial bleeding [9]. In addition, with the continuous-combined regimen, studies reported the lower the estrogen dose, the lower the rate of PMB. The administration of a lower estrogen dose revealed an estimated incidence of 20% contrasting with the 43% outlined by higher amounts of estrogen [10, 11]. On the other hand, the administration of progesterone or progestin without a previous or simultaneous endometrial exposition to estrogen seems not to result in bleeding abnormalities. Progestins differ widely in their chemical structures, pharmacokinetics, and potency [13] and are mainly administered to prevent endometrial hyperstimulation during MHT. Studies confirmed that progestogen molecules containing levonorgestrel, or medroxyprogesterone acetate (MPA), have a higher risk of developing endometrial hyperplasia than those containing norethisterone acetate (NETA) [14, 15]. In addition, considering the variety of combinations of estrogens plus progestins, Loh F.H. et al. demonstrated that women who received 1 mg E2/0.5 mg NETA had a better bleeding profile incidence (2%) than women who were administered 2 mg E2/1 mg NETA (23%) for 6 months [10]. Moreover, few studies supported better control of PMB during the administration of 1 mg NETA/5 mg E2 therapy compared to 0.625 mg CEE/5 mg MPA therapy in a 12-month follow-up [11, 16]. Thus, the incidence of PMB during MHT can be highly reduced by minimizing estrogen and progestogen doses while also choosing the proper compound combination. Some researchers noted that the interaction of specific molecules with the endometrium can explain the different incidences of PMB. However, the precise mechanism involved in bleeding abnormalities is still unknown. It probably results from multiple biochemical changes caused by the interaction of progestin plus estrogen with the endometrium. Archer et al. [17] studied biochemical changes during MHT using an immortalized endometrial cell line (Ishikawa). They observed that synthetic progestin, and progesterone to a lesser degree, significantly increased vascular endothelial growth factor (VEGF) mRNA and thrombospondin-1 (TSP-1). The imbalance in proangiogenic (VEGF) and antiangiogenic (TSP-1) factor seems to contribute to the angiogenic process and abnormal blood vessel formation, leading to a higher incidence of bleeding abnormalities. A schematic depiction of the effects of VEGF and TSP-1 level changes during MHT administration involving angiogenesis is shown in Fig. 1. However, more information on such bleeding abnormalities is needed, and the clinical implication of increased levels of VEGF after MHT administration, inducing abnormal bleeding, remains to be defined.

Fig. 1 Schematic depiction of the effects of VEGF and TSP-1 on angiogenesis involving new vessel and tube formation and elongation by mitosis and apoptosis [12]. The administration of progestins seems to have a significant role in increasing VEGF and TSP-1 levels. The alteration of proangiogenic (VEGF) and antiangiogenic (TSP-1) factors could cause angiogenesis disorders leading to irregular-shaped and abnormal superficial vessels in the uterine cavity of the progestin-only contraceptive uterus, highly notable during hysteroscopy [17]

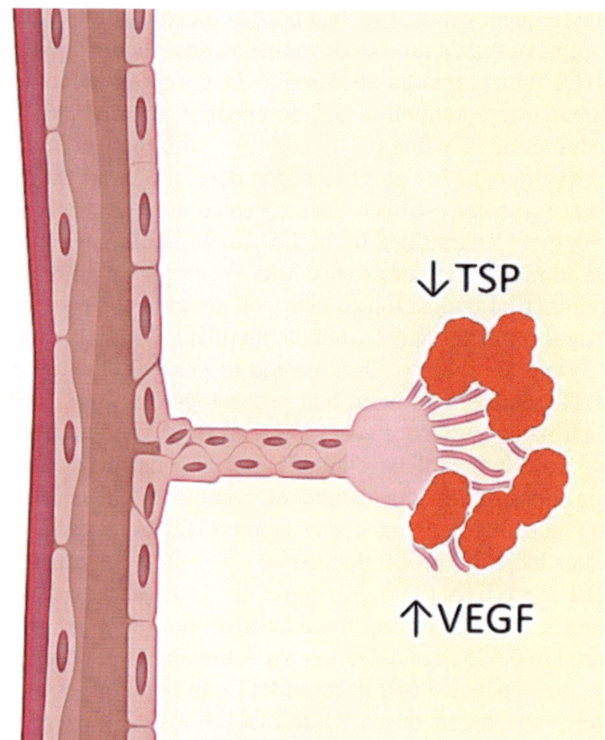

3 Any Proper Diagnostic Investigation During Postmenopausal Bleeding Abnormalities?

The causes of abnormal bleeding are characterized by different incidences depending on women's reproductive age, as shown in Table 1. The most frequent causes of abnormal bleeding during MHT administration include (1) poor compliance; (2) incorrect therapy administration, such as forgetting pills or concomitant use of antibiotics and altering compound absorption; (3) an unbalanced combination of estrogen-progestogen. Uterine pathologies are less common but more alarming causes of bleeding abnormalities and include (4) polyps, (5) endometrial hyperplasia, and (6) endometrial carcinoma. Thus, a proper diagnostic investigation is crucial to exclude severe endometrial pathologies while identifying the bleeding cause to allow for appropriate management and tailored treatment. Currently, there are no clinical guidelines on managing bleeding abnormalities during MHT. Therefore, there is significant variability in how providers perform diagnostic assessments. As a good clinical practice, diagnosis has to begin with a general evaluation including history and nature of bleeding episodes, associated symptoms, history of chronic or malignant pathologies, and administration of other medications, in particular contraceptives, non-steroidal anti-inflammatory drugs (NSAIDs), and warfarin or heparin [2]. In addition, a physical examination and a pelvic evaluation are always required, including speculum findings and bimanual pelvic assessment to investigate cervical or vaginal causes. Additional exams can also be carried out, including laboratory tests with a complete blood count and iron studies. Pregnancy testing and thyroid screening may also be appropriate. In addition, an evaluation of pelvic organs and endometrium has to be performed. Transvaginal ultrasonography (TVUS) is usually sufficient for an initial evaluation of bleeding abnormalities in postmenopausal women and a reasonable alternative to endometrial sampling [18]. In 2009 the Committee on Gynecologic Practice of the American College of Obstetricians and Gynecologists (ACOG) stated that when an endometrial echo less than or equal to 4 mm on TVUS is found, endometrial sampling is not required [19]. Nevertheless, not all uteri can be evaluated by ultrasounds, such as in cases of patients with myomas, previous surgery, obesity, and adenomyosis [2], as well as perimenopausal women who may not lend themselves to a meaningful ultrasound examination. In fact, in patients with the erratic estrogen production of perimenopausal ovaries, TVUS done at the end of a bleeding episode may be inadequate to measure endometrium thickness [20]. In all the cases previously mentioned, sonohysterography (SIS) may be crucial to virtually distinguish the presence or absence of actual anatomic pathology while also differentiate global versus focal changes [20]. As an alternative tool, hysteroscopy may undoubtedly be performed, although the issue of expense, operator dependence, and analgesia/anesthesia concerns. Endometrial biopsy is another assessment of AUB for evaluating the endometrium. Some studies promoted it as a standard of care in diagnosing PMB [21]. Others involved biopsy only after a diagnosis of cancer or atypical hyperplasia [22, 23]. In 2012 the ACOG stated, in their Practice Bulletin, that endometrial biopsy has "high overall accuracy in diagnosing endometrial cancer when an adequate specimen is obtained and when the endometrial process is global" [24]. Consequently, in clinical practice, an endometrial blind biopsy should not be performed due to its low sensitivity. Therefore, it is reliable in diagnosing global processes such as hyperplasia or carcinoma, if they occupy 50% or more of the endometrial surface. In summary, bleeding abnormalities during menopausal hormone therapy require investigation to exclude endometrial pathologies. Thus, in terms of endometrial biopsy, ACOG recommends it as a diagnostic end point only when a diagnosis of atypical hyperplasia or carcinoma is made because of its high false-negative rate in focal endometrial pathologies.

4 Conclusions

Postmenopausal bleeding is an important part of clinical practice for healthcare providers of women. The highest rate of bleeding abnormalities involves dysfunctional problems due to the administration of hormonal therapy. A reduction of bleeding episodes can be achieved by decreasing the dose of estrogen-progestin molecules. However, the precise mechanism involved in endometrial bleeding is not yet completely understood. Most of the time, bleeding is worrisome and negatively impacts patients' quality of life. Therefore, the goal should be to require prompt and proper interventions resulting in appropriate diagnosis and necessary tailored treatments.

References

1. Davis E, Sparzak PB. Abnormal uterine bleeding. Treasure Island, FL: StatPearls; 2022.
2. Goldstein SR, Lumsden MA. Abnormal uterine bleeding in perimenopause. Climacteric. 2017;20(5):414–20.
3. Moodley M, Roberts C. Clinical pathway for the evaluation of postmenopausal bleeding with an emphasis on endometrial cancer detection. J Obstet Gynaecol. 2004;24(7):736–41.
4. Abid M, Hashmi AA, Malik B, et al. Clinical pattern and spectrum of endometrial pathologies in patients with abnormal uterine bleeding in Pakistan: need to adopt a more conservative approach to treatment. BMC Womens Health. 2014;14:132.
5. The NHTPSAP. The 2017 hormone therapy position statement of The North American Menopause Society. Menopause. 2017;24(7):728–53.
6. Stefanick ML. Estrogens and progestins: background and history, trends in use, and guidelines and regimens approved by the US Food and Drug Administration. Am J Med. 2005;118(Suppl 12B):64–73.
7. Ziel HK, Finkle WD. Increased risk of endometrial carcinoma among users of conjugated estrogens. N Engl J Med. 1975;293(23):1167–70.
8. de Medeiros SF, Yamamoto MM, Barbosa JS. Abnormal bleeding during menopause hormone therapy: insights for clinical management. Clin Med Insights Womens Health. 2013;6:13–24.
9. Pan M, Pan X, Zhou J, Wang J, Qi Q, Wang L. Update on hormone therapy for the management of postmenopausal women. Biosci Trends. 2022;16(1):46–57.
10. Loh FH, Chen LH, Yu SL, Jorgensen LN. The efficacy of two dosages of a continuous combined hormone replacement regimen. Maturitas. 2002;41(2):123–31.
11. von Holst T, Lang E, Winkler U, Keil D. Bleeding patterns in peri and postmenopausal women taking a continuous combined regimen of estradiol with norethisterone acetate or a conventional sequential regimen of conjugated equine estrogens with medrogestone. Maturitas. 2002;43(4):265–75.
12. Archer DF. Endometrial bleeding in postmenopausal women: with and without hormone therapy. Menopause. 2011;18(4):416–20.
13. Stanczyk FZ. All progestins are not created equal. Steroids. 2003;68(10–13):879–90.
14. Hickey M, Ambekar M. Abnormal bleeding in postmenopausal hormone users-what do we know today? Maturitas. 2009;63(1):45–50.
15. Padwick ML, Pryse-Davies J, Whitehead MI. A simple method for determining the optimal dosage of progestin in postmenopausal women receiving estrogens. N Engl J Med. 1986;315(15):930–4.
16. Simon JA, Liu JH, Speroff L, Shumel BS, Symons JP. Reduced vaginal bleeding in postmenopausal women who receive combined norethindrone acetate and low-dose ethinyl estradiol therapy versus combined conjugated equine estrogens and medroxyprogesterone acetate therapy. Am J Obstet Gynecol. 2003;188(1):92–9.
17. Archer DF, Navarro FJ, Leslie S, Mirkin S. Effects of levonorgestrel, medroxyprogesterone acetate, norethindrone, and 17beta-estradiol on vascular endothelial growth factor isomers 121 and 165 in Ishikawa cells. Fertil Steril. 2004;81(1):165–70.
18. ACOG Committee Opinion No. 734 Summary: The role of transvaginal ultrasonography in evaluating the endometrium of women with postmenopausal bleeding. Obstet Gynecol. 2018;131(5):945–6.

19. ACOG Committee Opinion No. 440: The role of transvaginal ultrasonography in the evaluation of postmenopausal bleeding. Obstet Gynecol. 2009;114(2 Pt 1):409–11.
20. Goldstein SR. Use of ultrasonohysterography for triage of perimenopausal patients with unexplained uterine bleeding. Am J Obstet Gynecol. 1994;170(2):565–70.
21. Stovall TG, Photopulos GJ, Poston WM, Ling FW, Sandles LG. Pipelle endometrial sampling in patients with known endometrial carcinoma. Obstet Gynecol. 1991;77(6):954–6.
22. Larson DM, Krawisz BR, Johnson KK, Broste SK. Comparison of the Z-sampler and Novak endometrial biopsy instruments for in-office diagnosis of endometrial cancer. Gynecol Oncol. 1994;54(1):64–7.
23. Ferry J, Farnsworth A, Webster M, Wren B. The efficacy of the pipelle endometrial biopsy in detecting endometrial carcinoma. Aust N Z J Obstet Gynaecol. 1993;33(1):76–8.
24. Committee on Practice B-G. Practice bulletin no. 128: diagnosis of abnormal uterine bleeding in reproductive-aged women. Obstet Gynecol. 2012;120(1):197–206.

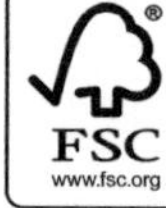

MIX
Papier aus verantwortungsvollen Quellen
Paper from responsible sources
FSC® C105338

If you have any concerns about our products,
you can contact us on
ProductSafety@springernature.com

In case Publisher is established outside the EU,
the EU authorized representative is:
**Springer Nature Customer Service Center GmbH
Europaplatz 3, 69115 Heidelberg, Germany**

Printed by Libri Plureos GmbH
in Hamburg, Germany